"Ditch the Drive-Thru!"

~ Successful Weight Loss for "Real Life" ~

By

Debbi Kennedy

The "Ditch the Drive-Thru!" Mom

~ Nutrition Education for a Future Generation ~

"Ditch the Drive-Thru!"

Successful Weight Loss for "Real Life"

Printed by CreateSpace
ISBN-13: 978-1497567627

First Edition

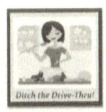

Table of Contents

Acknowledgements 4

Forward 6

Chapter 1   The "Cycle of Sabotage" 10

Chapter 2   The "Cycle of Success!" 16

Chapter 3   The "Nutritional Cliff" 22

Chapter 4   The Unknown 27

Chapter 5   Small Steps 33

Chapter 6   Sidetracked 38

Chapter 7   "Food for Thought" 44

Chapter 8   Insanity! 51

Chapter 9   "The Rules" 56

Chapter 10   Time-Saving Tools 75

Chapter 11   Starting Over 83

Chapter 12   Recipes and Extras 87

Chapter 13   A Final Thought 143

<u>"Ditch the Drive-Thru!"</u>

~ Acknowledgements ~

To my Parents, who always told me I have "so much potential"...

I finally KNOW what I want to do when I grow up! ☺

Thanks, Dad, for always encouraging me to "get my move on!"

Thank you, both, for your encouragement, love and support!

To my Kids and my Husband...

You make me want to be the best me I can be.

I am so blessed that God gave you all to me, and I love you!

To my dear friend, René...

You dragged me to that Half Marathon meeting that started it all!

You have listened tirelessly to my ideas, championed my dream,

encouraged my success, and helped keep me grounded

throughout this whole process. Thank you!

To Troy Vorse, Mr. "Web Guy Extraordinaire"...
You have continually worked behind the scenes to make
my website and online presence so successful!
I would NEVER be where I am today without ALL of
your hard work and incredible support! You rock!

To Tina Macuha and 'Good Day Sacramento' at CW31...
Thank you for allowing me the airtime that helped launch
"Ditch the Drive-Thru!" You have continually welcomed me on set
and given me the opportunity to reach people that
I never could have alone! You are the best, and I'm so grateful for
every opportunity I get to inspire your viewers! Thank you!

And last, but not least... To Erika, Erik, Ray, Geno, Victor, Richard,
and all the rest of the wonderful staff and volunteers at the
'Sacramento Food Bank & Family Services'...
You are truly the unsung heroes who work so long and hard to help so
many families continually "ditch the drive-thru", by providing fabulous,
fresh, healthy food, and nutritional resources in our community. I am so
blessed to partner with you in impacting families in such a positive way!
This is the very best thing I never knew I always wanted to do! ☺
Thank you, thank you, thank you!

"Ditch the Drive-Thru!"

~ Forward ~

I can't say I remember a specific time or day...

I just know I'd had enough!

I had just finished adding up the amount of money that we'd spent on eating out and I could have gone shoe shopping 14 times! I mean I could have gone shoooopping! For REAL shoes... not the "Buy One Get One ½ Off" kind! It was really ridiculous! 100's of dollars had been spent on fast food and restaurants within a matter of weeks! Granted, we'd been extremely busy that month, but good grief! If only I would've had some kind of a plan, or if I'd thought ahead just a _little_ bit about preparing our meals, think of all the money we could've saved!

I have been married for almost 20 years, and have struggled with weight for most of my life. (More about that later!) I am also the mom of two really great kids, a son and a daughter. We are currently at two different schools, and life is CRAZY!! I usually run in six different directions five days a week, and by the end of the day, I'm pooped! Between school, homework, hubby's job, church, sports, "Kennedy Cab Co." (Aka carpool), and everything else... "Stick a fork in me, I'm done!"

The more I talk with moms the more I hear the same theme: overworked, over-tired, over-stressed, overweight, and overwhelmed! The last thing we want to think about at the end of the day is having to make dinner for our family! Enter *"Ditch the Drive-Thru!"*

"Ditch the Drive-Thru!" is all about teaching you how to make a delicious, nutritious meal for your family in LESS time (and for less money) than it takes to go thru a drive-thru and pick up fast food. Really!

I am convinced that by the time you find your wallet or purse, grab your keys, get in your car, drive down the street, actually get your order in without WWIII erupting in your back seat, get your "correct" order home (good luck with that!), and shove 39 grams of fat down your family's throats... you can have a delicious, nutritious meal on your table that your family will eat and love! Less time, less money, less calories, and waaaay less fat! Don't believe me? It IS possible! Timer to table... less than 15 minutes! Really! And by the time you're done reading this book, you will be doing it, too!

"Ditch the Drive-Thru!" is about SO much more than just saving money. It's about saving our families! It's about saving memories! It's about "face time"... and I'm not talking about your iPhone!

> *~ It's time for us to take back dinner! It's time for us to unbury the kitchen table and use it for more than just homework! ~*

How many great memories do you have of your family dinners, and the time you spent laughing around the table when you were growing up? It's now just a thing of the past. Maybe you didn't have "family dinner" at your house and you just spent most evenings eating on TV trays in the living room. Either way, it's time for you to make it happen!

No matter how crazy life may get, we need to *make* time for family dinner. We only get one chance. We don't get do-overs!

The time is now! For yourself, for your wallet, for your waistline, and especially for your children...

It's time to "Ditch the Drive-Thru!"

Debbi Kennedy, Founder

Chapter 1

The "Cycle of Sabotage!"

Does this sound familiar? You close your eyes and step on the scale. With great anxiety and much reservation, you pry your eyes open, one at a time, and reluctantly peer toward your toes. Your dreaded reality is confirmed. You've gained weight... again. You look in the mirror, and it starts.

Disappointed and disgusted with what you see, you go to the freezer and grab the ice cream. You had *planned* to go out for a walk today, but now the only energy you have is to grab a spoon from the drawer and sink into your sofa with your favorite friend. *Today* was going to be different. *Today* was going to be a fresh start. "Oh well," you think, "I'll go for a walk *tomorrow*." And the "Cycle of Sabotage" begins...

Our nation is obsessed with food! We see thousands of commercials every year about what to eat, what not to eat, where to eat, when to eat, how much we should eat, and the list goes on... and on... and on! It's ridiculous! Nearly two-thirds of Americans are overweight! Everyone is looking for the next big thing in the diet industry. We want a quick-fix answer for a long-time problem! Everyone wants to know what the secret is to losing weight. What's the secret? What's the secret?! What's the SECRET??!!!

> *~ The truth is ... (spoiler alert) ... there is NO secret! There is NO magic pill, NO 'special sauce', and NO magic sprinkles! Eat less... MOVE MORE! That's it!* **Eat less of the bad, eat more of the good, and** <u>**move your body!**</u> *~*

I chose to start this book with this chapter on purpose! It is time for us to wake up! It is time for us to look at our weight and our heath *realistically!* There is no magic pill... there is NO secret, or quick fix!

Our <u>perception</u> is that if we can just find that one magic pill, or that one secret thing, then all of our weight issues will be magically cured! However, the <u>reality</u> is we must make one good choice at a time, day by day, that will lead us down the path to a healthier lifestyle and away from the "Cycle of Sabotage".

It dawned on me one day that I was stuck in an endless cycle of sabotage and self-defeat. Take a look at the picture below. It clearly depicts what I now call, "The Cycle of Sabotage".

THE CYCLE OF SABOTAGE!

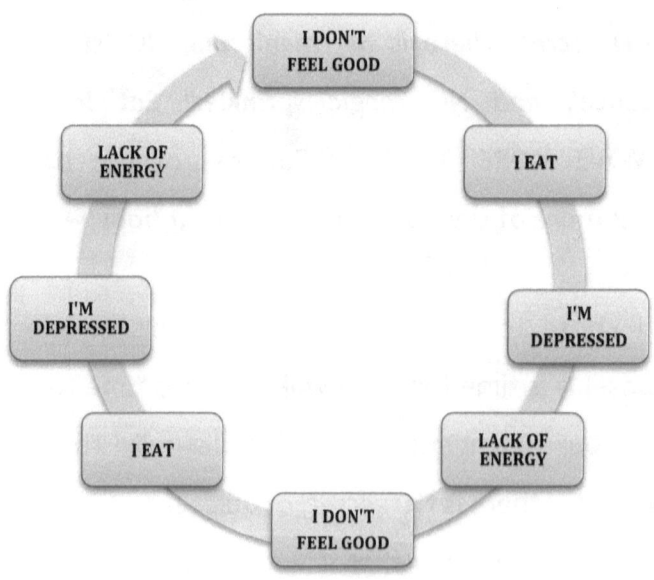

It always starts the same way with, "I don't feel good." I don't feel good, so I eat. When I over-eat, I gain weight, and I get depressed; when I'm depressed, I have no energy, so I certainly am not going to be motivated to exercise. When I lack energy, I don't feel good, so I eat more, which makes me depressed, which leads to more of a lack of energy, and here we are again... right back at the top where we started! Do you see how easily we can get sucked into this negative vacuum of self-sabotage? We can be our own worst enemy!

This book is not about a quick fix, or deprivation; it's about choosing a healthier way of life! It's not about "going ON a diet", because inevitably, if we go ON a diet, we will eventually go OFF a diet, and we wind up just riding around in circles on that merry-go-round of the "Cycle of Sabotage" again and again!

You do NOT have to give up everything you love to eat in order to be healthy. Don't tell me I can't have my carrot cake. "I loooove me some carrot cake!" I intend to eat it and enjoy every delicious morsel! Mmm... mmm... mm!! In fact, I love it so much I had to figure out a low fat recipe so I can enjoy it more often! You'll find it in the back of this book in the recipe section. Yummers! (Ok, now I want a piece, so let's move on! ☺)

You don't have to give up what you love to eat, but you do have to look at how _much_ you eat, and _why_. Are you eating because you are hungry? Do you eat because you're bored, or tired, or depressed, or angry, or hurt, or... any other emotional reason that pops into your head?

I have found that we need to examine _why_ we are doing things. (You'll have an opportunity to take some time to do that in just a few chapters.) Sometimes we may not know the "why", but if we are still willing to do the "what" in the meantime, the "why" will often be revealed down the road, and we'll feel a whole lot better along the way!

If you are living in the detrimental "Cycle of Sabotage", my prayer is that you will find hope within these pages.

> _~ You are **NOT** defined by your fat! You are uniquely special, and you were created with a purpose that only you can fulfill! ~_

If you are still breathing, God is not done with you, and you were put on this planet for a reason!

> *~ Get out of your own way! Give yourself a break. Stop the negative words, stop the self-loathing, stop the excuses, and stop the "Cycle of Sabotage!"~*

You CAN do it, and you _will_ see results when you begin making positive choices to break this cycle in your life. Only then will you begin to experience SUCCESS!

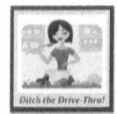

Chapter 2

The "Cycle of Success!"

We spend way too much of our lives living in the downward spiral of the "Cycle of Sabotage"! As you can see from the previous illustration, it is a never-ending circle of depression, guilt, and self-defeat. So how do we break this cycle? How do we change our thinking? I'm so glad you asked! ☺ I call it, "The Cycle of Success!"

The "Cycle of Success" begins in the same place... "I still don't feel good!" However, the difference between sabotage and success is what we do with our next step! In order to break the cycle of self-defeat and depression, I must make a *different* choice at Step #2...

> *~ Instead of choosing to eat, I choose to MOVE! ~*

THE CYCLE OF SUCCESS!

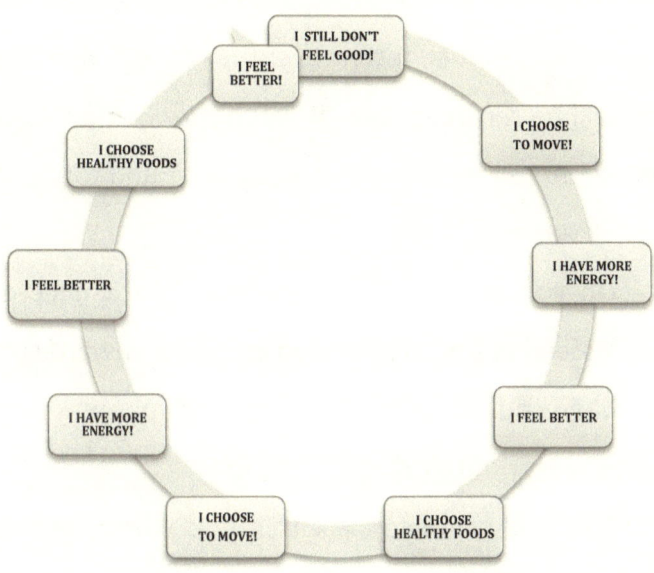

The "Cycle of Success" starts in the same place: "I still don't feel good, and I still don't like the way I look!" (Same initial problem.) BUT... instead of choosing to eat, I choose to go for a walk. I CHOOSE to be active and MOVE my body!

When I go for a walk and move my body, those little endorphins kick in, and I have more energy! When I have more energy, I feel better!

When I feel better, I make better food choices! When I'm eating healthier foods, I want to move! When I move, I have more energy, and I feel better, which makes me want to continue to choose healthy foods, and I continue to feel better! Eventually the "I don't feel good" will be replaced with "I feel better", and "Voila!" We have broken the "Cycle of Sabotage" and found the "Cycle of Success!"

Do you see the difference that ONE choice can make? Instead of getting trapped in the downward spiral of sabotage and self-defeat, we can "act" our way into a whole new way of thinking... SUCCESS!

This was never so clear to me as when I decided to train to walk a Half Marathon with the American Heart Association in 2012! Yes, that is 13.1 miles, and I walked every one of them!! My much thinner "friend" (and I use that word loosely) decided that she wanted to train to walk a Half Marathon, and she thought that I should do it with her. HA!

I was a size 24/26W at the time, about 150 pounds overweight, and I pretty much thought that she was out of her ever-lovin' mind! (Sidebar... If you don't have a friend like this, find one!) I told her that I would go with her and "support her", but I knew there was just NO way

I could realistically train to walk 13 miles in 13 weeks!

When we went to the information meeting, there were several people who stood up to give testimonials about their prior Half Marathon experience. One man had Diabetes and had one leg that was shorter than the other. Ok, he was pretty convincing. Then, our soon-to-be, new "hero" got up and spoke.

An 80 year-old man, who had heart transplant surgery, had walked this Half Marathon the year before! (Really?! That's what they're gonna throw at us?! Not fair!!) He was amazing, and so inspiring, and I looked at both of those men and thought, "What's my excuse?! I then looked and my friend and asked, "What's our excuse?"

I signed on the line that night and committed to walk! And you know what? It was one of THE best decisions I've EVER made... NO regrets!! We trained, we walked, and we finished! In fact, we trained, we walked, and we finished _again_ the next year! Can I get a "WooHoo!"?!

The main thing that impressed me, aside from their step-by-step training program, is that not once did they ever obsess about food! Not one time did I ever hear anyone say, "Oh, you can't eat thaaat!" In fact, food wasn't ever even a focus until we had our class on "Fueling the Athletic Body" when we got up around 6 miles in our training! This was fascinating to me!

Every other program or 'diet' that I've ever tried _always_ started with the _focus on food_! It was always "eat this and don't eat that", and counting this, and measuring that... and totally obsessed with the food! This program only said, "Move your body!" Just walk!

As I began walking, I began to feel better, and I had more energy. Slowly but surely, week after week, the pounds and inches started coming off! I began to see positive, _measurable_ results, and a light bulb came on for me during those weeks of training!

> **"I am absolutely convinced that if our country would become LESS obsessed with food, and MORE obsessed with healthy exercise, we could see an end to, or at least a dramatic decrease in, obesity, diabetes, heart disease, high cholesterol, high blood pressure, and so many other ailments that are plaguing our overweight nation!"**

When we start with exercise, everything else falls into place! That's why I call it, "The Cycle of Success!"

Merriam-Webster's Dictionary defines the word 'success' as, "the correct or desired result of an attempt." I believe that the most "successful" people in life are NOT the people who never fail... they are the ones who simply *never stop trying!* They are unwilling to give up, and they *continue* to attempt to reach their goals until they achieve their desired results!

One of my favorite quotes, by Robert Collier, says this: "Success is the sum of *small* efforts repeated day in and day out." This has encouraged me many times over the years, especially when I don't feel like I'm making much progress in my life, or I'm not seeing the desired results that I'd like to see!

"Reality TV" constantly shows us unrealistic pictures of remarkable weight loss transformations in a matter of weeks, however, in the midst of the busy-ness of "real life", successful weight loss does NOT happen overnight! I have to remind myself that "success" WILL come as long as I continue to make good choices, day by day, and break the "Cycle of Sabotage" once and for all!

When the "blahs" hit and I don't feel good, I can either choose to *eat* and *feel worse,* or I can choose to *move* and *feel better!* We have an opportunity to make choices everyday... Choose <u>SUCCESS!</u>

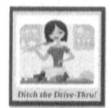

Chapter 3

"The Nutritional Cliff"

You couldn't turn on a TV or radio in December of 2012 without hearing the phrase, "Fiscal Cliff". Certain tax rates that were previously in place were getting ready to expire by January 1st, and our entire nation was faced with bills that we couldn't afford to pay! Our nation, as a whole, was heading right over a financial cliff that would cause major economic devastation from which we would not soon recover.

I find it very interesting that no one has yet to equate the "Fiscal Cliff" of America with the "Nutritional Cliff" of America. *Well, let me be the first!*

> **"We, as a nation, are heading straight towards a 'Nutritional Cliff' in our country!"**

According to the 'US Centers for Disease Control and Prevention 2010 National Health and Nutrition Examination Survey', "Nearly 36% of adults and 17% of children are obese – meaning they have a body mass index (BMI) above 30." To translate, this means that approximately 1/3 or _more_ of their total body weight is made up of _FAT_!

This calculates to a total of 50% among adults and children in our country! Of all the men, women, and children in the United States, one out of two is obese! And let me just clarify; this is NOT including all the people who are "overweight"! With those numbers added in, we land closer to 70% of America dealing with weight issues! 7 out of 10! We are standing at the edge of a Nutritional Cliff, and if these numbers don't change, we are going to head straight over the edge!

Have you ever watched the "Price is Right"? I LOVE the "Price is Right"! You cannot watch that show and be in a bad mood! Even the people who don't win are still so happy, just because they've been on the show, and they get to "spin the wheel"! It's great!

One of my favorite games is "Yodely Guy", as Drew Carey has affectionately named him. The game is the same as all the others... guess the right price and win the prizes! This game, however, holds the fate of one very cute, Swiss yodeler who will fall over the edge of the cliff if the numbers are off.

Up, up, up he goes with his yodeling music blaring, blissfully ignorant of the fate that awaits him, should his newly selected contestant friend be incorrect! The contestant guesses the price of an item, and "Yodely Guy" heads up the hill, one line for every number that is incorrect. The audience shouts and applauds, and many times gasps, when "Yodely Guy" plunges over the edge and the game is done. Aaaaaahhhh.

That's the picture I have in my head. Our blissfully, ignorant country, yodeling along our merry way, oblivious to the "Nutritional Cliff" ahead and the devastating fate that awaits us!

> *~ I am absolutely amazed that with such an extreme obesity problem in America no one is shouting about our 'Nutritional Cliff'! Well, I am SHOUTING! I am yelling at the top of my lungs, "LOOK OUT! We're headed for the edge!!" ~*

It has been estimated that in the year 2009, nearly 5 billion dollars was spent on cholesterol/statin medications alone! (This number fell from 10 billion in

2005, but only because using generic drugs, rather than name brand, cut this cost dramatically!) According to the Associated Press, nearly 320 BILLION dollars was spent on prescription drugs in the year 2011! 320 BILLION! Can you hear me NOW?!

We spend more time in the drive-thru than at the dinner table, and we are eating fried foods as one of our main food groups! Physical Education, recess, and sports programs have been cut from schools. School days are longer, playtime is shorter, and loads of homework and technology have become the primary focus, encouraging a more sedentary life-style. Is it *any* wonder our kids are struggling to be healthy?!

Statistics show that nearly one in three children born in the year 2000 are likely to develop Diabetes. 1 in 3! It has also been said that this is the first generation of children that is on track to NOT outlive their parents! This is *unacceptable!*

~ *DO YOU SEE THE SIGN YET ???* ~

Warning... *"NUTRITIONAL CLIFF AHEAD!"*

We MUST be the voice of change! WE must be the ones to take a stand and say, "No more! Not in my house, not in my school, not in my neighborhood, or my state, or my country, or my world!" WE are the ones who hold the power to 'change the nutritional environment of our homes'!

Parents, listen up! WE are the ones who do most of the grocery shopping, WE are the ones who buy the food and bring it home, WE are the ones who drive the car through the drive-thru, WE are the ones who don't know how to say, "NO" to our whiny little two year olds when they want sugary, 'dessert' cereal for breakfast...

and WE are the ones who have the power to change it!

We may not be able to stop the "Nutritional Cliff" of our country right now, but we can certainly take some small steps to keep our family from going over the edge!

The time is NOW! For yourself, for your wallet, for your waistline, and especially for your children...

It's time to "Ditch the Drive-Thru!"

Chapter 4

"The Unknown"

How long have you been overweight? (If you've never struggled with this, I envy you!) I think the last time I remember being a healthy, "normal" size was probably when I was a kid. I've always had a "large frame" for my size. I have large bones and broad shoulders. Beautiful... if you're a Size 6 and 5'9"! I'm not... never have been!

Although I was a 3-sport athlete, and in fairly good shape throughout my Jr. High and High School years, I always seemed to be one of the biggest girls on the team, and I always felt like I wore the largest uniform.

I remember, once in high school, going dress shopping with our choir for an upcoming choir concert and not being able to buy a certain dress for our group, because they didn't have an XL that fit me. Embarrassing and depressing!

I also remember talking to my friend about my frustration of being the "biggest one" in the group! Looking back now, I know I wasn't that big... I think I was about a size 12/14? Yet somehow I always felt "fat". I was very outgoing, confident, cute, and had a lot of friends, so I never really let my "size" get me down, but it was always there.

When I went off to college, I gained my "Freshman 15"... and never lost it! In fact, it multiplied. Up and down, up and down, but mostly up. Since then, I've mostly been heavy.

When I got married in 1994, my wedding dress was a size 22. When this book was written, I was wearing a size 18/20 jeans. However, I was as large as a size 26/28W (3X/4X) when I was my heaviest after kids, and as thin as an 8/10 for a short time when I'd lost a bunch of pounds after my college days. I tell people, "I have been up and down the scale more times than a concert pianist! You name it... I've tried it! I have 'been there, done that', and I've got 14 t-shirts in 8 sizes that don't fit!" ☺

My point is that I've known what it's like to be overweight for most of my teen and adult life. It's just the way I am... it's what's familiar. This has been so much a part of my life that I don't really know anything else, and I wonder sometimes if the fear of the unknown is the thing that keeps me from breaking out of the "Cycle of Sabotage"?

I'm not a Psychologist, but I have learned a few things about human behavior in the past years of dealing with my "stuff". (That's a WHOLE other book, by the way!) One of the things I've learned is that many times we say things with our words, but we tell a whole other story with our actions!

> ~ *Many times in life we may think that something is true, and we may even convince ourselves to believe it. However, our actions tell a whole other story!* ~

I have to confess, I am the 'poster child' for this... guilty as charged! I call it "Perception vs. Reality".

It dawned on me one day that I was living in a "perceived reality". By that, I mean I had a view of my life that was not grounded in reality. It is very easy in the chaos and 'busy-ness' of life to lose sight of what is actually going on around us! We get into our groove and we think that our life is a certain way when it actually could be the exact opposite, we just don't realize it.

We need to wake up and look at our life for _what_ it is, _where_ it is at the time! My 'perception' is... "I _want_ to do this..." however, the 'reality' is... "I can _actually_ do this..."

I find this to be especially true for mothers of young children. I certainly found it to be true with me when our kids were little! We want to continue to do what we've always done without missing a beat. We get sucked into the "perception of perfection" and feel that we need to be the "perfect" Mom, _and_ wife, _and_ employee, _and_ school volunteer, _and_ team mom... _and everything else_ in our crazy, busy lives!! When the reality begins to set in that we may have to give up some of things we've been juggling for years, it can be very easy to slip into feeling like a failure.

My perception may be that I _want_ to go to the gym and work out 5 days a week. However, in the midst of "real life" – diapers, naps, and Cheerios in the couch – the reality might be that I just need to pop in a 30-minute workout DVD while my little angels are napping ... AND BE OK WITH THAT!

With all of the technology, videos, DVDs, and apps that have come on the scene in the past decade, you can get a fantastic workout without ever having to leave your living room or step foot inside a gym anymore! Personally, I LOVE 'Zumba Core' for the Wii and Xbox 360! 20 minutes burns about 200 calories! WooHoo!!

My point, again, is this: I have to be willing to look at my life for _what_ it is... _where_ it is at the time. _'Not now'_ doesn't mean _'not ever'_, it just means _not right now_, during _this_ chapter of my life. I have to be realistic about the time that I _actually_ have, and I need to stop beating myself up over the things that I'm NOT doing!

Would you pleeeeze give yourself a break and stop beating yourself up for who, and what, you're NOT?! You are MORE than the number on the scale or the size tag on your jeans. Let me repeat that, just in case you missed it! You are SO much more than the number on the scale or the size tag on your jeans! Do NOT let those numbers define you!

There is a 'Special K Cereal' TV commercial that I love! It shows various women getting measured for jeans in a fitting room. None of them look very excited to see what the tape measure will reveal. However, when they look down to see the words, "Beautiful"... "Inspirational"... "Confident"... instead of their measurement _size_ number, their whole countenance changes, and they begin grinning from ear to ear!

It completely changed their perception of themselves. I love that!

I was watching the 'American Comedy Awards' one night, and I heard a quote that I just had to share! When the famous and incomparable comedian, Bill Cosby, had finished a story about one of his first stand up routines that completely "bombed" on stage, he had this to say about fear: "You have to show up! You _cannot_ allow yourself to talk yourself into being so scared of who you are... because _you_ are the _only_ person who can represent who _you_ are!" *(Thank you, for that, Mr. Cosby!)*

You can choose to settle and talk yourself out of "showing up", or you can work towards becoming your very best self! Don't you deserve to be your _best_ self?

> *~ **None of us know what tomorrow will bring. Don't allow the fear of the unknown to keep you trapped where you are now, and don't let it keep you from getting to where you want to go!** ~*

Where you are right now is NOT where you always have to be... **IF** ... you decide that you WANT to change it, AND you take the steps to MAKE it happen!

Chapter 5

"Small Steps"

Let me start this chapter by saying, "Small steps forward are still moving in the right direction!" All too often in life we get wrapped up in large gestures and grandiose ideas. We get trapped in the thinking that if it's not a huge step forward, it doesn't count. Wrong!

> *~ Even small steps forward are still moving in the right direction! ~*

I have found, throughout most of my years, that it's really not the big things that trip me up. It's the little, insignificant things that tend to cause me the most grief. I don't really struggle with the huge indiscretions, like lying, cheating, and stealing, but I do find I tend to have a very difficult time with being consistent in the daily grind of life.

I get very frustrated with myself when I don't see huge strides made, cause I always _knew_ that by the time I hit 40 that I would "have it all together"! Right. Then I get completely overwhelmed feeling like there is so much I still have to do (or "fix") that I don't even know where to begin! The pounds I still need to lose, the house I never manage to completely de-clutter, and the financial hill that we just can't quite conquer are all overwhelming if I try to tackle them all at once. However, if I am willing to continue to take small steps in the right direction, I will eventually find success.

Again, it's what I do with "Step #2" that determines the cycle that follows. Am I going to sabotage myself with the negative thinking and self-defeat that comes with believing that only the big steps count? Or am I willing to quell the negative voices and choose to be faithful in the seemingly "insignificant", small, steady steps that will eventually lead me across the finish line?

We've all heard the story of the "Tortoise and the Hare". This cocky little rabbit seems to have it all together. He's slick, he's quick, and he's moving right along with huge leaps and bounds, until he gets sidetracked and decides that he has time to slack off.

Mr. Tortoise, on the other hand, just keeps moving. (He reminds me of Dory, from the Disney movie 'Finding Nemo', who sings, "Just keep swimming, just keep swimming... swim, swim, swim!") Yes, he's slow, and his progress is nothing compared to his quick-footed opponent, but he keeps moving forward! In the end, his determination pays off and he wins, what seemed to be, an impossible feat! Why? Small steps!

> ~ **Even small steps forward are still moving in the right direction!** ~

It was a beautiful January morning. The air was crisp and the sun was out for the first time in a week, so I decided to take a few minutes and prune some of our bushes by our front walk that were in desperate need of attention. When our neighbor across the street said, "Good Morning!" and asked how I was doing, I replied, "Not bad for a Monday. I figure I can't do miracles, but I can do something!" As I reached into the bush and pulled out the left over cobwebs that our son had used to "decorate" for Halloween (did I mention it was January?!), that thought struck me like a TON of bricks!

> *"I may not be able to do miracles today, but I can do something!"*

Small steps! If only I would've taken some of that advice and made a little time each week to pay attention to our bushes, our yard wouldn't look like an over-grown weed farm! A few minutes a day, or even a week, would have made a huge difference!

The same is true with weight loss. It's so easy to get frustrated with ourselves because we don't see the huge numbers drop on our scale like on "The Biggest Loser". We get sucked into the "Cycle of Sabotage" and think that losing "only one pound" isn't significant, but let's stop and think for a moment...

If you were to walk 20 minutes a day, 6 days a week, you would walk about 6 miles a week. The average person can walk a 20-minute mile, at a pace of 3mph. (I'm 5'4" and I can walk a mile in under 20 minutes.) If you walk 6 miles a week, that adds up to 24 miles every month, and you would have walked approximately 312 miles by the end of a year! That's the equivalent of walking nearly 12 Marathons in 365 days! (Math... when will I use this? You're welcome!)

By the way, that's the same distance as walking from Sacramento, CA to the top of the Grapevine in Southern California heading to LA! WHAAAT???!! Think about that! Oh, and get this! By the end of one year you would have burned approximately 31,200 calories! How's *that* for math!?

My point is this: Small steps matter! Do NOT allow yourself to get sucked into the "Cycle of Sabotage", and do NOT allow yourself to think that if you don't go run a Marathon it doesn't count. It counts! Small steps count!

So you're not going to lose 100 pounds and 5 dress sizes by the end of the year... would you like to be 20 or 40 pounds lighter, and 1 or 2 sizes smaller, rather than staying in the same place you are right now? Small steps forward are still moving in the right direction!

> ~ *It's the small, steady steps everyday, in <u>every</u> area of life, which will eventually get you across the finish line to where you will finally find success!* ~

Remember, "Success is the sum of small efforts, repeated day in and day out." Small steps count! Take your first step today...

"GET YOUR MOVE ON!"

Chapter 6

"Sidetracked!"

Confession time: I have spent a good deal of my life being sidetracked. (A really, whole lot, whoppin' good deal!) In fact, I would say that I am THE self-declared, "Queen of Unfinished Projects"! I am absolutely faaabulous at starting projects! If you need your troops rallied for some big event, or you need someone to get everybody fired up for a cause, I'm your gal! Yes indeedy, I'm a <u>great</u> project starter... just NOT such a great project finisher!

I always have the best intentions, but somehow that doesn't quite seem to be enough to carry me through.

> *~ All too often in life we rely on our good intentions to carry us through, and all too often we just wind up disappointed! ~*

The problem with good intentions is that they are downright unreliable. Our good intentions can often be overshadowed by the current crisis of the day, or simply derailed by a fleeting fancy that catches us off guard during a distracted moment. We mean well, but somehow that list we intended to accomplish becomes a distant memory by the end of the day.

After many years of watching my name slip down "my list" day after day after day, I decided that my name needed to go on the top, and STAY on the top! Now, that may sound selfish to you, especially if you are a mom, but I can tell you from personal experience that unless YOU put YOUR name at the top of YOUR list, no one else WILL!! We are SO great at taking care of everyone, and everything, else around us, that we wind up letting all those other 'more important' things crowd our name off of our list. No good!

The number one rule to keep me from getting sidetracked is for ME to keep MY name at the TOP of MY list! I realize this seems selfish, however, personal experience has proven again and again that if I don't take care of me, _no one else will!_

I am the keeper of my health – mentally, spiritually, emotionally, and physically – and if I don't MAKE the time to nurture each one of these areas, I will not be as effective in nurturing those around me. Sure, I can get by for a while, but eventually something's going to give. It's sort of like skimping on sleep. We may be able to fake it for a while, but when we try to continue to get by with less sleep than we need, usually we just 'crash and burn'.

I have found that it can be hard to get started with an exercise program. When to work out, how to work out, and where to work out, are all obstacles that must be overcome in order to be successful. I've also found that it's often harder to 'stay started' and continue in my new habit once my schedule starts to catch up with me, or my life gets in the way. I get sick, the kids are out of school, we go on vacation, or I just don't have the 'gumption' today to get my rear end out of bed today... whatever the reason... I get sidetracked!

I am SO not a morning person, and I used to drive right back home after dropping my kids off at school, just counting the minutes until I could crawl back into bed and 'hug my pillow'! "I'll go to the gym _tomorrow_ morning", was always my excuse. Yet somehow tomorrow never came. Good intentions, nevertheless, sidetracked... again... and again... and again!

In order for *me* to be successful, I had to change my entire morning routine! My new Monday through Friday school year schedule now looks like this: I get up in the morning and put my swimsuit on under my clothes when I get dressed. I eat a light, healthy breakfast, and I have my coffee. (We have our priorities, you know! ☺) Then I brush my teeth, grab my swim bag, and drive my kids to school. As soon as I drop them off at 7:30am, I drive *straight* to the gym around the corner to hit the pool by 7:40 for 45 minutes of laps. As long as I stick to my schedule, I'm great!

Quite frankly, life is full of excuses! In fact, here's another confession: I had a lot of trouble keeping my workouts on the top of my list during the holiday season! We had a *really* cold couple of weeks, the kids were out of school, we slept in later, and I wasn't up, and dressed, and out the door like my usual early morning, scheduled (*key word!*) routine. I now know that I need to re-think this and create a new plan for next time so I can avoid slipping back into the "Cycle of Sabotage".

It's all too easy to slip back into old habits! It's not like I 'fell off the wagon', or 'went on a bender' to binge eat myself sick, or that I even intentionally decided NOT to go to the gym... I simply got "sidetracked" and let myself fall back into my same old rut. I found myself thinking that I would feel better if I could 'just get caught up on some sleep', and I'd be _sure_ to get back to the pool the next day!

Those few days turned into weeks, and the funny thing is that after a few weeks of excuses and missed workouts, I certainly didn't feel any better, or more rested! I just felt fatter, lazier, and more tired... and quite honestly, I was pretty disappointed that it seemed so easy to slip after all the amazing progress I'd made in the previous months! I MEANT to get to the pool, I had very _good intentions_ to get to the pool, but it just didn't happen. What did happen? Well, as I see it, two things:

#1) I didn't keep MY name at the top of MY list! I didn't stick to my schedule, and I let everyone and everything else become a priority. Not that the other things aren't important... they just have to be kept in perspective.

#2) I wasn't accountable! I didn't have a "workout buddy" to cheer me on, or to check in with me when I didn't show up. Having a set place and time to exercise with a specific person helps you both stay on track! Put it on your calendar and block out that time just for YOU! It's a great way to build a friendship and get fit together!

There are many free fitness groups you can join, as well. "Find what you love, and do it!" Check out your local walking or running clubs, find a biking group, or take a Yoga class. Finding other people with similar fitness interests and goals will help you stay on track!

> ~ If we're not careful, all of our excuses... "I can't", "I don't want to", "I don't feel like it", or "I'll do it tomorrow"... become the thing that derail us day after day, and keep us from becoming the person that we really want to be! ~

I found that when I stopped making excuses and started putting MY name on the TOP of MY list, I finally saw results! When life gets crazy, and my schedule gets full, I have to remind myself of this again and again!

If you've gotten sidetracked, <u>TODAY</u> is the day to get back on track! Take a look at your schedule. What's changed? What's different? Where did you get derailed? Don't beat yourself up! Just stop the excuses, put your name back on the TOP of your list, and get back on track! You CAN do it...

"Get Your Move On!"

Chapter 7

"Food for Thought"

Before we move on, I'd like you to take a few moments and think through the questions on the following pages. I'm going to encourage you to actually write out your answers. You can copy these pages and fill in the blanks, or you can write your answers on these pages in the book. You could also choose to use another piece of paper, or a journal. Whatever you decide, keep it somewhere handy so that you will be able to refer to it again in the future.

> ~ *Be honest, and be 'real' with yourself during this process. There are no wrong answers.* ~

Take some time to think through each of these questions, one by one. Make sure that you allow yourself plenty of time and a quiet place, free from distractions.

If you feel stuck on a question, that's ok. Simply move on to the next one, and then come back and try to answer that question at the end. Usually, when you begin writing things down, you begin to find answers that you may not have known were there all along.

What thoughts or ideas stand out the most to you in the pages you have read?

_____

_____

_____

_____

_____

_____

Where do you feel your name falls right now on your list of priorities and things to do in your life, and why?

_____

_____

_____

_____

_____

_____

_____

Have you been (or are you now) stuck in the "Cycle of Sabotage"? Explain.

_____

_____

_____

_____

_____

_____

What do you think keeps you from breaking this cycle in your life, and why? What do you need to do to change it?

_____

_____

_____

_____

_____

_____

_____

What do you think needs to happen in your life for you to finally experience the "Cycle of Success"?

_____

_____

_____

_____

_____

_____

_____

_____

The following questions are here to help you think through your current schedule and set some realistic, achievable, "real life" exercise goals!

<u>How</u> are you going to "Get Your Move On!"?

Be specific! For example... "I will walk for 20 minutes a day,

4 days a week."

☐ Walk ☐ Jog ☐ Run ☐ Aerobics ☐ Water Aerobics
☐ Swim ☐ Bike ☐ DVD ☐ Other

_____
_____
_____
_____
_____
_____
_____
_____

<u>When</u> are you going to "Get Your Move On!"?

Be realistic! If you're not a "morning person" (like me!), DON'T

set a goal to get up at 5am!

_____
_____
_____
_____
_____
_____
_____
_____

<u>Where</u> are you going to "Get Your Move On!"?

Again, be specific! For example... at the gym, on a treadmill, walking outside with a friend, DVD, etc.

_____
_____
_____
_____
_____
_____

What are your weight loss goals? Explain.

□ Lose weight □ Build muscle □ Get stronger
□ Increase energy □ Improve heart health
□ Improve sleep □ Lower blood pressure
□ Lower cholesterol □ Start training for an event
□ Find a new sport □ Other

_____
_____
_____
_____
_____
_____

Think of the family and friends in your life. Who will support your weight loss goals, and be a workout partner?

_____
_____
_____
_____
_____

What, if anything, do you need to do to "change the nutritional environment of your home"? Explain.

_____

_____

_____

_____

_____

_____

_____

Picture yourself in one year... who do you want to be, how would you like to look, and what do you want to be able to do? (I want to be a size smaller and walk a 5/10K!)

_____

_____

_____

_____

_____

_____

_____

Picture yourself in 5 & 10 years... who do you want to be?

_____

_____

_____

_____

_____

Hopefully now you have a little clearer picture of where you are, how you got here, and most importantly, where you want to go! I would encourage you to revisit these questions again during your weight loss journey. You may find that some of your answers change as you see the pounds come off!

I tend to be the kind of person who needs my toes "stepped on" every once in a while, so having something like this to help me take a good, hard look at what I'm doing is very helpful. I hope it helps you, too!

It has been said that the most successful people in life are the ones who actually write their goals down on paper, so keep this in mind...

> *~ Whether it's in your personal life, school, work, business, or anything else, having a written plan will help you to be much more successful! ~*

Set your goals, write down your goals, refine your goals, and refer to them often! It can be very empowering to see your dreams written out in 'black and white', and it also serves as a continual reminder of whether or not you are on track to finally get to where you want to go! *Keep on keepin' on!*

Chapter 8

"Insanity!"

Have you ever heard the 'unofficial' definition of insanity? Insanity is... "Doing the same thing over and over, but expecting different results." Does that ring a bell for you? It sure does for me! If I were being honest I would have to say that I've been riding the 'insanity roller coaster' for the majority of my life!

I'm very quick to tell people, "I am not an organized person, I just play one on TV!" I'm sure that there are people who've seen my little TV segments and think I am SO organized and I have it all together... WRONG! Not at all! In fact, that's one of the reasons I created my monthly "Mix 'n Match Meals" Menu Plan, and the main reason that I wrote this book!

(By the way, shameless plug... You can download your own menu at www.ditchthedrive-thru.com!)

I was sick and tired of spending money on food that was wasted, and I was really disgusted with hitting the drive-thru every week because I didn't have a plan! Talk about insanity!

I don't know where I originally heard it, but one of my all time favorite quotes is this: "If you always do what you've always done, then you'll always get what you always got!" Profound right? I've also heard this variation that I like even better!

> **"If you always do what you've always done, then you'll always <u>be</u> what you've always <u>been</u>!"**

Remember when we talked about the "Cycle of Sabotage"? We wind up going around in circles in a downward spiral because we keep making the same lousy decisions! So here's something to ponder... if we keep making the same lousy decisions, why in the world do we think that somehow we will wind up in a different place? We seem to think that if we just keep doing the same thing over and over, somehow, magically, we'll wind up with different results. It doesn't work that way! We have to make a *different decision* to get a *different result!*

So now what? Well, my friend, there are certain times in life when we all reach a pinnacle point. We have an "epiphany", a "light bulb goes on", or we "come to our senses"... any of which lead us to a defining moment when we have to decide, "Now what?" Well, now the choice is yours. You get to choose whether or not you are going to continue in your insanity, depression, and self-defeat, or if you are going to start over.

My guess is that I probably haven't really told you anything you don't already know... you just needed to hear someone else confirm it! Maybe you are hearing some of this information for the first time, or maybe you've heard it before and you chose to ignore it. Whatever the case, you now have a choice. YOU are in control of your next step!

You can put this book down and decide to go back to what you were doing before, but I'm guessing that what you were doing before probably wasn't working for you, or you wouldn't be reading this book! (Hey, I call 'em like I see 'em! ☺)

The choice is yours... the time is now! *Today* is the day you choose to start over. *Today* is the day you get your fresh start! Your new "diet" does NOT start on Monday... your new *day* starts <u>TODAY!</u>

There are as many books on diets and weight loss as there are foods on the earth! They are countless! I have seen countless numbers of books telling the stories of people who've lost hundreds of pounds! "She used to be a Size 26 and now she's a size 2!" or "He used to weigh 400 pounds and now he's a Triathlete!" It's very easy to find a 'been there, done that' book. Don't get me wrong... that's really great for the ones who have been successful with the 'before and after' books! However, my whole goal with THIS book is to give you the '<u>during</u>'!

> *"I want to motivate you to get started, and I want to encourage you to keep going! I want to inspire you to 'change the nutritional environment of your home', and I want to cheer you on as we work towards being fit and healthy... TOGETHER!"*

I am NOT an "expert" in this field, and I certainly have not yet arrived! I still have a long way to go to finally reach my weight loss goals. I am not a Nutritionist; I am not a Doctor, or a Health Professional in any health field of any kind.

What I am, is an ordinary, *determined* woman who has found, mostly through trial and error, the keys that have helped me begin to shed my extra pounds. One of those keys is this:

> **"Know what works, and do what you know!"**

Will there be setbacks? Absolutely. BUT... I know what works, and if I continue to do what I know, I know I will reach my goals... one day at a time, one step at a time!

I used to say, "Eat less... Move more!"

Now I simply say this:

"MOVE YOUR BODY!!"

When you start to move your body, and you start eating more of the good, you'll want to eat less of the bad... and you WILL be successful!

My hope Is that you have found some encouragement within these pages, and that you have been inspired to make some changes in your life! You CAN get off the weight loss merry-go-round once and for all, and you CAN start living a healthy lifestyle! And, yes, you CAN have your cake and eat it, too... just in smaller pieces! ☺

Chapter 9

"The Rules"

I have to confess that I don't tend to be a real "by the book" kind of gal. I tend to think that if something comes with directions, they are to be referred to only if I get stuck. (This drives my husband crazy, by the way!) However, as we have already seen, when left to my own devices, I can make a real mess of things!

I don't tend to really have "rules" per say, but I have definitely found that following these "Ditch the Drive-Thru!" guidelines have helped me stay on track. When I have a plan and follow "the rules", I tend to stay much more organized, and I find that my grocery dollars go much further!

You will find all of "The Rules" at the end of this chapter, but I thought I'd take the time to walk you through them one by one.

Rule # 1 ~ Cook Once, Eat Twice!

If you're going to go to all the trouble of pulling everything out to make dinner, you might as well maximize your efforts by making extra portions that you can use later in the week or freeze for later in the month. This is a great way to save time and stretch your dollars. It works for breakfast, lunch, and dinner!

Skillet meals are my favorite, super simple, "Cook Once, Eat Twice" meals to make. My 'Very Veggie Scramble' is a fast and easy way to ensure a delicious, nutritious breakfast for the entire family in just a matter of minutes! Make a whole skillet full and then put the extra portions into the fridge in single serve containers, so they can be pulled out for a quick breakfast later in the week.

The $5.00 Family Skillet, and other pasta and meat skillet meals, are a great way to maximize your cooking efforts and "mix 'n match" your meat from one meal to the next! For example, if you buy a 20 oz. package of lean ground turkey, cook it all at once, but use ½ for your spaghetti sauce and the other ½ to make our "Lucky 7 Chili". Cook once... Eat twice!

Rule # 2 ~ <u>Use Your Microwave</u>

If you don't have a microwave, get one! If yours is broken, fix it, or get a new one! This is absolutely THE fastest way to save time when you are trying to get dinner on the table quickly! It will cut your cooking time in half or more, depending on what you're making. Plus, in the hot, summer months you won't have to heat up your house by using your stove... an added bonus in our neck of the woods when it's a balmy 105° outside!

Let me just add my 2¢ here, if I may? Occasionally I am asked questions about "killing the nutrients in food" when using a microwave. From what I have read, I have come to this conclusion: If we are starting with fresh, nutritious food, and steaming it for just a few minutes in the microwave, I do not believe that we are doing that much damage to the food. Besides, even if we "kill off" some of the nutrients in fresh broccoli, for example, I still believe it is MUCH more nutritious than most of the food you will find in any drive-thru!

Rule # 3 ~ <u>Keep Your Fridge and Pantry Organized</u>

I am the worst offender of this... especially when life gets crazy! There's nothing that makes me angrier than having to throw out perfectly good food that went bad, because I forgot about something tucked away in the back of my fridge! Those veggie drawers at the bottom?! Ugh! They can be a terrible, lonely place for fruit and vegetables to die if we forget about what's down there! Take a few extra minutes each week to clean your fridge and pantry, and check for expiration dates. This helps with meal planning and eliminates the excuses to hit the drive-thru. It also gives you room for new items when you find them on sale!

Rule #4 ~ <u>Stock Up On Sale Items</u>

I am a "couponer"! I was introduced to couponing years ago, and the light bulb went on! I figured out how to save 100's of dollars every month by using coupons and buying things on sale. My friends have referred to me as, "The Coupon Queen"! If you are a couponer, great! If not, I would encourage you to learn how to use coupons. By the way, you don't have to be "extreme" to cut your grocery bill significantly! Just using your "digital coupons" from your local grocery store cards can save you hundreds of dollars a month without ever having to clip anything!

Whatever you decide, make sure that you buy extra items you use when they go on sale. Things like whole grain pastas, a variety of sauces, canned beans and tomatoes, and frozen veggies are especially on my list of "must haves" to use when I want to throw dinner together really quickly!

Rule # 5 ~ Stock Up On Quick, Lean Protein

Keeping quick fixin', lean protein on hand is a great way to ensure a healthy, balanced meal in a hurry. My favorites are frozen chicken tenderloins or thighs, thin cut pork chops, canned beans, chicken, and tuna! These are all shelf stable ingredients that will last a while in your pantry, or meat that can be easily kept in your freezer. Since meat is usually the most expensive part of a meal, stock up when you find it on sale! Remember that thawing it out will save you a TON of time preparing dinner. Pull it out of the freezer and put it in the fridge so you won't have to wait for it to defrost.

Rule # 6 ~ Always Have Frozen Veggies

There has been a long-time debate as to whether or not frozen veggies are as nutritious as the fresh ones. Depending on where you live, they can actually be fresher! Frozen veggies are picked, washed, cut, packaged, and frozen right away, as opposed to the travel time that it may take those same veggies to get to your local supermarket.

My first choice is usually fresh, but the frozen steamer bags are a perfect way to get those veggies on the table in no time at all! Most bags steam in the microwave in about 4 minutes! Throw one in while you're finishing your main dish, and you'll have a completely nutritious meal.

~ I've included my "Top 10 Veggies & Fruit" list at the end of this chapter! There are SO many fruit and vegetables with SO many great nutrients... but, if I had to choose, these are all extremely versatile and mostly available all year. Plus, I can "mix 'n match" them for snacks and meals all throughout the day! Deeelicious! ~

Rule # 7 ~ <u>Always Buy Low Fat</u>

Whenever you have an option, always buy low fat, especially when it comes to dairy products! Nearly all milk products – yogurt, cheese, cream cheese, cottage cheese, and sour cream – now come in a light version. If you are concerned about extra calories, and you are drinking whole milk, stop it! Unless you are extremely mal-nourished, you do not need to be drinking whole milk! Switch to 2% - *yesterday!!* If you are drinking 2% and trying to lose weight, think about switching to 1%. Trust me, your pallet will adjust, and you will save a huge amount of calories and saturated fat.

I do not advocate going completely nonfat! We <u>need</u> fat in our diet. That's one of the things that help give us shiny hair and soft skin, and it is vital for brain function, memory, and cell growth and development! Studies are showing more and more that Omega-3 fatty acids are vitally important when it comes to brain function. Just remember that we want the bulk of our fat to come from things that grow from the ground, NOT animal fat. Animal fat and animal by-products contain higher levels of saturated fat, and that's the fat that can tend to clog the arteries.

Here's a silly little poem I wrote to help me remember what kind of fat to eat:

"If it grows from the ground, then scarf it down!
If it swims in the sea, then it's for me...
(And that's where I find Omega 3!)
If it walks on 2, then some will do...
But if it walks on 4, once a month and no more!"
(Hey, I warned you it was silly!)

"*If it grows from the ground*"... it's good fat! Avocados, nuts, seeds, and oils that come from plants, like Olive Oil, all contain essential, heart-healthy fats needed for brain function and tissue development. They tend to be most beneficial when eaten in their raw state.

"*If it swims in the sea*"... Fish is a great way to find those essential oils that your body needs. Fish oil contains heart-healthy, Omega 3 and Omega 6 fatty acids. These not only help your heart, but also keep your hair and skin looking beautiful, and aid in brain function! One side note... be careful of the amounts of mercury that can be found in some fish. Wild caught is always best, and canned sardines are a great source for good oil! Try them on crackers for a snack in the afternoon.

"If it walks on two"... Chicken and turkey, and other fowl, are lower in saturated fat and also contain higher amounts of monounsaturated fat, which tend to be higher in Vitamin E and help fight off cell-damaging chemicals in the body. They also contain polyunsaturated fat, which helps with brain function and tissue growth.

"If it walks on four"... This can be a tricky subject, and there are as many different opinions as there are 'experts' in the world! For me, beef is my last option when it comes to fat. Pork tends to be lower in fat, but I still eat it less than chicken or turkey. Since animal products tend to contain higher levels of saturated fat per serving, I try to limit them in my diet.

Like everything else, I won't tell you not to eat it, but I will suggest that you limit it. A nice, small steak once or twice a month probably won't kill you, but once or twice a week is probably not so great for your heart.

Something to consider, however, is that red meat does contain iron, which is often lacking in women. Dark leafy greens, leeks, asparagus, and beets can all add extra iron into your diet if you need it, or you can also add a vitamin/nutrient supplement if your numbers are really low. Consult your doctor for more information.

I used to drink my calories! If I were to add up all the additional calories that came just from coffee, soda, juice, and everything else in a day, I could have easily added an additional 500+ calories in <u>one day</u>! *Easily!!* As much as I love my "Large, Extra Hot, Non Fat, 6 Pump, Gingerbread Latte with Light Whip, Light Foam", I might as well have bought a big piece of carrot cake, and eaten the whole thing!

Specialty coffees and other decadent drinks can be dessert in a glass, but we don't tend to count those calories in our minds, because we're technically not "eating them". What's worse, I am convinced that the food we consume in our cars does NOT register at all in our brains! Calories are calories, and they ALL count! Just because you're not chewing, doesn't mean it doesn't count!

> *~ I cannot stress this enough:*
> **READ, READ, READ YOUR LABELS! ~**

Juice and soda are _extremely_ high in calories and sugar! Eat an apple instead of drinking apple juice. Try sugar free mix-ins instead of soda. This is extremely important for our children! Get them into the habit of drinking water!

Order your coffee as a treat once a week, and use your coffee pot at home! Shake up some "fru-fru" flavored coffee creamer to make it frothy, and pour it in your coffee to make a "Lazy Latte"! Save the fat, calories, and expense of the drive-thru every morning!

You will be _amazed_ at the amount of calories (and money!) you can save just by decreasing sugary drinks and increasing water! One question: How do you know if you are drinking enough water? Simple... your pee should be clear. No joke! If you are drinking enough water and you go to the bathroom, you shouldn't really see anything when you are done! Now, there are times when certain supplements or medications will change the color of your urine, but other than that, the goal is clear! ☺

Rule # 9 ~ Watch Your Portion Sizes!

I think that this is one of the biggest areas where people can really pack on the pounds. It takes 20 minutes for your stomach to tell your brain that you are full. 20 minutes! Most people have eaten their entire plate of food and are finishing their second plate by the time 20 minutes is up!

I cannot stress HOW critical it is that you SLOW down when you eat! Chew your food thoroughly. Chew each bite 20 times before you swallow... put your fork down in between bites... use your opposite hand to eat... whatever trick you need to help you slow down when you're eating, do it!

If you scarf down your first plate of food in 10 minutes and then start on a second plate, by the time your stomach says that it's full, it's too late! You've already eaten 2 full meals! Believe me, if you multiply all those calories in a year's time, you will not like what the scale has to say! Watch your portion sizes!

By the way, restaurants are the biggest offender of this! Most serve enough for two people on one plate, so we eat way too much food in one sitting! Plan to ask for a box at the _beginning_ of your meal and put half away for later, or just split a meal when you go out to eat. Your wallet and your waistline will thank you!

The same is true when it comes to snacking... watch your portion sizes! DO NOT just open a box or bag of your favorite chips, flop down in front of the TV, and start eating! It's all too easy to scarf down waaay too many calories and not even realize you've eaten them! _Read your labels_, and count out a serving. Yes, I said it... "Count your chips!" ☺

I heard someone once say, "Use a salad plate for dinner, and a dinner plate for salad!" I thought that was a great tip, and I try to keep that image in my head when I'm dishing out my meal portion sizes.

> **"Always remember... Eat when you're hungry, _stop when you're NOT!_"**

We have always been taught, "Eat when you're hungry, stop when you're full", right? What's the problem? The problem is that by the time you are feeling "full", you've already eaten too much! Stop when you are no longer hungry, and you will feel much better in the long run!

Rule # 10 ~ _"Get Your Move On!"_

This has become my motto... "GYMO!" I used to do the "gym thing" and work out, but I was never very consistent. I swam for a while, and LOVED it, but our gym membership just got to be too high with only using it a few months out of the year, so we gave it up.

Then I found walking... and biking... and Wii Zumba Fitness! You do NOT have to spend hours in the gym to be healthy and get results! _Find what you love, and do it!_

One of my favorite things to do is walk! If you can walk from your door to your car to go to work, you can walk! Get off the couch and commit to 20 minutes a day, 6 days a week. This way, if you miss a couple days, you'll still be moving a good portion of the week! You will be amazed at how great you will start to feel, and studies are beginning to show that walking can actually add years to your life... what more incentive do you need?

I was having pretty severe pain after I walked my second Half Marathon, so I went in for an X-Ray. Unfortunately, I found out that I have severe Arthritis in my right ankle, and I also had a small fracture at the time! The cartilage is mostly deteriorated, and there's just not much that can be done at this point. The

Podiatrist told me that my next Half Marathon needed to be on a bike, so I started biking... and swimming! I decided to start swimming 6 days a week at the gym! (I don't mind paying for it when I'm actually using it!)

Since then, I try to swim laps for about 50 minutes a day, 4 – 5 days a week, and do additional Water Aerobics classes during the week to work out different muscles.

I also continue to get out and WALK! I don't do the miles like I used to, but it is still great exercise! I walk the 5K now instead of the Half Marathon, but remember... *Small Steps Count!* The pounds and inches are coming off, and I feel better and stronger each week! I've found some new muscles, and I can even do pushups!

My point is this: it would have been very easy for me to have a pity party about my bum ankle and stop exercising, but I didn't! I started biking when I was in a boot for 5 weeks, and then I swam with a neoprene brace on my ankle for a month, using mostly my upper body!

I made the choice to "show up". I decided that I was going to get fit and healthy, and work towards being my best self! I made a decision to "Get My Move On!" and change my life, and I found ways to make it happen... one day at a time!

Get Your Move On!" (GYMO!) Find what you LOVE, and do it! Walk, jog, run, bike, swim, do Zumba, Step Aerobics, or Yoga, play tennis or racquetball, try rowing or kayaking... the possibilities are endless!

> *~ When you exercise, you feel better, when you feel better, you want to eat better, when you eat better and are exercising, you will have more energy, and you WILL find the "Cycle of Success!" WooHoo! ~*

Rules to Help You "Ditch the Drive-Thru!"

1. Cook Once... Eat Twice!
Use ingredients for more than one dish, and make extra portions to be used later in the week.

2. Use Your Microwave
Cooking in a microwave can cut your time in ½! (I also recommend buying a Pasta Boat!)

3. Keep Your Fridge and Pantry Organized
There's nothing worse than having to throw away perfectly good food because it's gone bad! Keep track of your ingredients and clean out your fridge weekly.

4. Stock Up on Sale & Pantry Items
Buy extra items you use when they go on sale so you can pull them out at a moment's notice.

5. Stock Up on Quick, Lean Protein
Keeping quick fixin', lean protein on hand is a great way to ensure a healthy meal in a hurry.

6. Always Have Frozen Veggies
When possible, fresh veggies should be your first choice but, when you're short on time, steamer bags or frozen bags of veggies are a great way to get your "Daily 5"!

7. Always Buy Low Fat

You can save a huge amount of calories and fat by buying 2%, 1%, and especially nonfat dairy products.

8. H2O is the Way to Go!

You can cut thousands of calories by replacing one sugary drink a day with water! Water also helps flush out the toxins in your body, and helps you feel fuller throughout the day.

9. Watch Your Portion Sizes

Remember... it takes 20 minutes for your stomach to tell your brain you are full!

10. "Get Your Move On!"

Get off the couch and move! When you start exercising you feel better, and you will naturally want to eat better. GYMO!

"Ditch the Drive-Thru!" Top 10 Veggies & Fruit

1. Mini Sweet Peppers ~ Just 3 have 270% Vitamin C!

2. Ruby Red Grapefruit ~ Lots of Vitamin C,

   and Pantothenic Acid helps boost metabolism!

3. Yams (Sweet Potatoes) ~ Vitamin A & Fiber

4. Bananas ~ A great source of Potassium!

5. Soy Beans ~ Fiber and Protein for a quick snack on the go!

6. Spinach ~ Vitamin A and Iron

7. Onions ~ Vitamin C

8. Blueberries ~ Full of Antioxidants!

9. Avocados ~ Heart Healthy Fat & Vitamin E

10. Mushrooms ~ Vitamin D

"Nutrition-and-you.com" is a comprehensive, user-friendly, website that I use as a reference. It has complete nutrition information for lots of fruit and veggies, along with nuts, seeds, herbs, and spices. It is extremely helpful!

Chapter 10

Time Saving Tools

The following pages are included to help give you a jumpstart on getting meals on the table. These are a few tips and tricks that I have used to help me get organized, stay on track, and save money!

People always ask me if I have recipes available. I try to post a "Recipe of the Week" on my website, www.ditchthedrive-thru.com, under the "Recipes" Tab, about once a week. While I do try to provide easy recipes that are readily accessible, I don't currently have a cookbook. I mean, really… have you been to Barnes and Noble lately? If you can't find a cookbook that you like out of the 1000's on the shelves, I would politely suggest that you just might be too picky!

> *"I am much more committed to teaching people cooking concepts rather than just providing recipes to follow. My feeling is this: Give a man a fish, and he eats for a day. Teach a man to fish, and he can make Fish Tacos for the rest of his life!"* ☺

I want you to be successful in creating meals in your kitchen, and one of the things I have learned over the years is that having the right tools makes a huge world of difference in saving time and preparing meals! Being able to chop and prep veggies quickly makes your job a whole lot easier! And, the easier things are to use, the more likely we usually are to use them, right? *Here are the "must have" tools in my kitchen:*

1. A Microwave!

If you don't own a microwave, get one! If yours is not working, get it fixed! My microwave is my absolute #1 time saving tool in the kitchen! It's not just for reheating your coffee anymore! C'mon, people! Love your microwave, use your microwave, become friends with it, and it will not disappoint you. You can cut your cooking time in half and get dinner on the table more quickly!

2. A "Pasta Boat"!

The 'Pasta Boat' is a fabulous microwave pasta cooker (refer back to #1!) that cuts your cooking time way down! Originally these were "As Seen on TV" only, and could be yours "for the incredible low price of only $19.95+S&H!" Now you can find them at many local discount stores, or even local thrift stores, if you're really lucky! I found one for only $3.00! Bar-gain!!

3. A Four-Inch 'Santoku' Chef's Knife

The right knife can make all the difference when you are trying to get things done quickly. I have fairly small hands and have found that the 4 or 5 inch Santoku knife with a rubber grip handle works very well for just about everything I need to do. It chops, it slices, and it's very versatile! If it's possible, try a knife out in your hand to make sure it has a comfortable grip. It will make a big difference by the time you're done doing all that slicing and chopping! By the way, take time to practice your knife skills. You can learn a lot by watching your favorite foodie TV shows!

4. A Knife Sharpening Steel

There is nothing worse than trying to slice a tomato with a dull knife! By the time you're done, you might as well have just used tomato juice! Having a sharpening steel in your drawer can be a huge help to keep your knives sharp and in good condition. If you don't know how to properly sharpen your knives, ask your butcher to show you the next time you're in your supermarket meat department.

5. A Large Cutting Board

Having a good work surface is really important when you are prepping your meals. Invest in a good cutting board. I have one large wooden one and several sizes of the plastic ones. That way, I'm covered no matter what I'm doing, and I don't have to take time to wash my board in the middle of preparing my meal.

6. A Good Large 12-Inch Nonstick Skillet

I LOVE my "veggie pan"! I have a large, 12-inch, nonstick skillet that works great for sautéing all of my veggies! You will notice I didn't say, "An expensive nonstick skillet". You do NOT need to spend a lot of money for any of these products. In fact, it's a great idea to check around at your local thrift stores. Many times you can find great products that have been gently used at a fraction of the cost!

7. A Large Nonstick Chicken Skillet w/ Glass Lid

I find that I use this skillet more than my veggie pan when I cook chicken because it has straight sides and it just seems to hold more meat. The glass lid is always nice just so you can keep an eye on your meat when it's cooking.

8. A Good Small 8 or 9-Inch Nonstick Skillet

Again, it does NOT have to be expensive. A little olive oil in the bottom of a good nonstick pan will go a long way. I use my smaller skillet for my veggie scrambles and eggs in the morning. It's also my "must have" pan for my crepes!

9. A Large Stockpot

I love soup! I think it's one of the easiest, most nutritious, meals you can make really quickly. A good quality, enamel coated, cast iron stockpot is a great way to get all those veggies in one pot, with leftovers. Cook once, eat twice! ☺

10. A Crock Pot

A Crock Pot or slow cooker is a "must have" for any busy mom. It is a HUGE time saver and will yield a very large meal for a very small amount of work. I have the 3-in-1 that comes with 3 different sized bowls, which offers a great variety for whatever I want to cook!

11. A Mandolin (Not the musical kind!)

Find some sort of a slicing mandolin that you can use to thinly slice veggies quickly. This tool makes things go much faster when you are trying to prep meals. If you practice your knife skills, it's fairy easy to cut or slice practically anything in no time, but a mandolin is still great!

12. A Medium Size Colander (Strainer)

You need to have a good colander that you can grab to rinse all those veggies that you'll be cooking! If you get a "Pasta Boat", the lid locks and strains. Brilliant!

13. Good Storage Containers

Last, but not least... it is *really* important that you spend a few dollars on good, airtight storage containers for your pantry, fridge, and freezer.

Remember that "Ditch the Drive-Thru!" Rule #1 is "Cook once, eat twice", so you need to have good storage containers around to make sure those extra portions don't go to waste.

Also make sure that your flour, sugar, and other pantry staples are sealed up tightly to stay fresher longer. Check your local thrift stores for great deals on Tupperware brand containers. They keep all those delicious veggies crisp and juicy, too!

Please note... nowhere in that list did you hear me say, "expensive"! You do NOT have to spend a lot of money to get good quality kitchen items. There are all kinds of kitchen gizmos and gadgets that you can waste your money on, but there are very few you actually need to make a great meal in your kitchen. I think this list is a great start to help you "Ditch the Drive-Thru!"

I am <u>very</u> quick to tell people, "I am not an organized person; I just play one on TV!" I am VERY guilty of having waaay too much stuff in my kitchen! I have found that once my kitchen is over-cluttered it is very difficult to find the motivation to clean it up just so I can cook dinner and mess it up again! So, once more, the drive-thru becomes a very tempting offer!

De-clutter your kitchen (she reminds herself, again!) and stick with the basics.

> ~ *Keep it simple! You can make a delicious meal with one skillet, one burner, and a microwave. It doesn't have to be fancy, just effective.* ~

If you find that it's not working the way you want, try something else! The most important thing is that you just keep at it until you find the things that work best for you and your family. You'll be SO glad you did!

Chapter 11

"Starting Over"

Did you ever play 'Four Square' as a kid? I loved the game, 'Four Square'! I've always been a bit competitive by nature, so I was pretty good. Inevitably, there was always that one kid that had to have a "do-over". Either the ball was on the line, or it was too close to call, or they just weren't ready when the game started... whatever! There were 12 different reasons they had to have a "do-over"!

There have been many times throughout my life that I would've liked a "do-over"! Several things come to mind: getting my college degree, spending more time with people I love before they are gone, and mostly, getting a handle on financial issues in my life when I was younger so I could have avoided some of the disasters I've had to endure!

I've often wished that my life had a "remote control" and I could just rewind back to right before I really messed it all up. This way I could have the chance to do it differently and wind up with a better outcome. Obviously this is NOT the way that life works. We don't get "do-over's"!

As I've mentioned, I am not an organized person. In fact, not only am I NOT organized, but, sadly, my disorganization has caused my family a great deal of stress over the years. I cannot tell you the amount of times that I have wished that Fairy Godmother of mine would show up with her magic wand, and pull a "Bippity Boppity Boo!" on my clutter!

I used to watch TLC's show, "Clean Sweep". You know, the show where they go into someone's messy home, pull out everything in it, sort it all out, get rid of everything they don't need, and then give them a "Bippity Boppity Boo" with their magic wand... *all in just 48 hours!!* I was always SO inspired and SO motivated, until I looked around at my clutter and felt helpless to even know where to start!

As our kids have gotten older I've watched them struggle with keeping their rooms tidy and neat, like any other kid, so we've continually tried to encourage them and give them the tools they need to help them conquer this area. I do NOT want them to struggle with this like I have!

When our daughter's room finally had too much stuff, I told her that we were going to work together as a family and do a "Clean Sweep" on her room. At first she was anxious, thinking that we were just going to back up a dump truck and load it all in! But after explaining to her how we would pull it all out, and sort it into 'give', 'throw', and 'keep' piles, she paused and said, "I guess I can start over." Such wise words from a 10-year old!

I would love to tell you that we were able to do a miracle in her room that weekend and we've _never_ had another messy day since. Not so. Just like everything else, we have to keep working at it... one day at a time.

The same is true with life. Occasionally, life get's "messy", and it's when the mess of life tries to creep back in that sometimes we just have to go back to 'square one' and start over.

Generally speaking, nothing good in life comes easily. We have to work hard at changing the things that are important to us, and then keep working in order to see the results that come from the changes we've made.

Everyday we have an opportunity to start over. I don't care if you have been fat your whole life, you can start over! You can start moving... TODAY! If you don't feel that you've been a good example for your children, you can start over... TODAY! If you have been living in the "Cycle of Sabotage", you can start over! You can break the cycle... TODAY! It's _never_ too late!

> *~ If you woke up this morning and you are still breathing, you can start over! The last chapter of your life has NOT yet been written. You, and you alone, decide what your next step will be! ~*

You can continue to make excuses for what you haven't done, and continue to wallow in self-pity and regret, or you can begin to take the positive steps that will change your life and lead you into the "Cycle of Success!" The choice is yours...

The time is NOW! For yourself, for your wallet, for your waistline, and especially for your children...

Its time to *"Ditch the Drive-Thru!"*

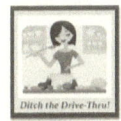

"Ditch the Drive-Thru!" Recipes

Even though this is not a cookbook, I wanted to include some of my favorite "go to" recipe ideas that I use when I need a quick and easy meal.

I think there are a lot of people that tend to rely too much on specific recipes. It's very important to me to focus on teaching cooking 'concepts', because I want you to be able to make these dishes for yourself again and again.

I've included a variety of meals for breakfast, lunch, dinner, and dessert, to give you a starting point and some inspiration to get cooking! I've chosen specific recipes that will show you the concept of preparing a certain type of meal, and all the recipes are designed to feed a family of four, usually with leftovers for lunch the next day.

You can find these full color recipes and much more at www.ditchthedrive-thru.com under the 'Recipes' Tab, and you can LIKE our Facebook Page, as well, to keep up with more delicious, nutritious information!

Enjoy, and Happy Cooking!

Very Veggie Scramble

There is NO doubt about it... breakfast truly IS the most important meal of the day! It affects my entire day... from how I feel in the morning, to how hungry (or cranky!) I am in the afternoon, and all the snack choices that I make in between.

One of my favorite morning breakfasts is my "Very Veggie Scramble"! It costs just pennies to make, takes only a few minutes, and it is chocked FULL of vitamins, nutrients, antioxidants, and enough protein and calories to keep you satisfied until snack time or lunch! Set aside a few extra minutes in the morning for breakfast and I think you'll see the difference it makes! Enjoy!

Ingredients

- **Eggs, or a carton of egg substitute**
Egg Beaters, or "Just White"' are great, too!
- **Any veggies you have on hand and like!**
We want COLOR... we eat with our eyes first!
Onions, sweet peppers, zucchini, broccoli, mushrooms, and spinach are my favorites!
- **English muffins, bagels, or wheat toast**
I like the "extra crispy" English muffins!

Directions

- Heat a nonstick skillet to med/hi with 1 tablespoon of olive oil.
Spreading the oil around the pan with a rubber basting brush before it gets hot is a great way to use less oil!
- Put 1 English muffin in the toaster per person.
I use a toaster oven, so I can do them all at once! They need about a good 5 minutes in my toaster oven to really get crispy.
- Chop onions and add to pan; sauté for about 2 minutes.
- If you are using whole eggs, crack 2 eggs per person into a large bowl, add a splash of water, and scramble 'til frothy.
- Chop the rest of your veggies and add them into pan in order of "hardness"... broccoli and peppers would go in before mushrooms and spinach.
- Cook the veggies for about another 2 minutes.
- Scoot all the veggies to one side of the pan and pour in about half of your scrambled eggs.
- Push the eggs around the pan until they start to set.
- When the eggs in the pan are almost set, pour in additional liquid eggs and cook until set, but still wet.
- When eggs are done, stir the veggies around with eggs to combine and serve immediately!

Serve with a crispy English muffin or toast, and a "Lazy Latte", and enjoy knowing you're getting your family's day off to a great start!
Put any leftovers in the fridge for later in the week!

"Benny Biscuits"

If you've ever ordered Eggs Benedict in a restaurant, you know it's delicious! What you may NOT know is that they are NOT low calorie at all! And forget about trying to recreate them at home, unless you have 'egg-cellent' egg poaching skills! ☺ (Buy an extra dozen eggs so you can practice! Just sayin'...)

Not only does it take 45 minutes on average to prepare, it is FULL of fat and calories! Traditional Hollandaise Sauce basically goes like this:

Take 10 tablespoons of fat, add 3 more blobs of fat, add salt to the fat, and then stir and cook, stir and cook, stir and cook! Way too much time for the morning rush, and did I mention the <u>FAT</u>?!

To prove my point... Here's the breakdown of the fat and calories from a well-known pancake house! Whaaaaaat??!!!!

Calories	Fat	Carbs	Protein	Sodium
1020	58g	78g	43g	3,190mg

Seriously... YIKES!!

So... for anyone who wants the 'Eggs Benedict' experience without all the fat, calories, and time-consuming precision, I have the answer! "Benny Biscuits"!

I am not kidding when I tell you that this is one of my all-time favorite breakfast sandwiches!! It is SO fast, and SO yummy! These do not have Hollandaise Sauce, but when you bite into that runny yoke, you won't even miss it!

They are done in about 6 minutes, and waaaaay less fat, calories, and expense than ordering in a restaurant! Not only that, it's a sandwich (albeit a messy one!), so you can take it with you on the go if you're really pressed for time! Just make sure to grab an extra paper towel to take with you for a 'bib' in the car... trust me, you're gonna need it! Enjoy!

Ingredients

- **1 English muffin** (the 'Biscuit')
- **1 large egg**
- **2 pieces thinly sliced (honey) ham lunchmeat**
- **Butter** – just a little to spread on the biscuits
- **Fresh Spinach** - Optional, but HIGHLY recommended! ... You'll see! It's grubbin'!
- **Salt and pepper**
I use Season Salt and Garlic Pepper! SO much flavor... so little sodium!
- **Olive oil or pan spray...** so your eggs won't stick.
A tiny egg pan or silicone egg rings are helpful!

Directions

- Put English muffin into the toaster and toast until crispy, somewhere between 3 & 5 minutes.
- Heat a small egg pan to medium heat with 1 teaspoon of olive oil.

Spread the oil around with a basting brush to cover the bottom of the pan before it heats up.

- When the pan is hot, gently crack one egg into pan, trying to keep the yoke in the center.
- Season with salt and pepper.

- Watch your egg closely! As soon as the egg white turns white and sets up, it's time to flip it over.
- GENTLY flip it over so you don't break the yoke... but don't worry if you do, just scramble it instead!

(Using a small silicone spatula will help!)

- Immediately add 2 slices of thin ham lunchmeat on top of the egg. Use 1 slice if it's thicker ham, or you can also use Canadian Bacon.
- If you are adding spinach, add a handful and spread out on top of the ham slices, keeping it in the center.
- Take the pan off the heat and turn off the burner... unless you're making more!
- When the English muffin is done, spread a small amount of butter on each biscuit.
- Holding the pan in one hand, place one biscuit on top of your egg "benny", and carefully flip it over onto the biscuit.
- Place it on your plate & top with the other biscuit.

Be prepared when you hit the middle... that oozy goozy yoke is gonna run all over, but it's so good when you get to sop it up off the plate. Deeelicious!

Carrot Cake Mini Muffins

It's no secret that I LOVE Carrot Cake! Unfortunately, it's also no secret that it is nowhere near low fat!! Eggs, oil, sugar, cream cheese... delicious, but yikes! We MUST remedy this! Immediately!

There is another recipe on our website for 'Quick and Easy Pumpkin Muffins' that are made with one box of cake mix and one can of pumpkin. Really simple and really yummy!! A good start, but can we do better? I think we can!

I volunteer with the Sacramento Food Bank and Family Services, doing live cooking demonstrations for the clients who attend their Mobile Food Truck Community Distributions. One of the produce items one week was bananas, but they were really ripe and needed to be eaten quickly. Everyone was asking about a Banana Bread recipe, but we didn't have one to share.

After coming home, I decided that I needed to come up with an easy, deeelicious, low fat muffin recipe that could use bananas in place of the fat and oil. I also wanted to "veggify" them, of course, but still have them taste delicious! Let me just say, "Mission accomplished!!"

So, the next time you're craving a really yummy muffin or piece of cake, don't spend extra money on extra fat and calories. Make these at home instead... your family, your wallet, and your waistline will ALL thank you! Enjoy!

Ingredients

- **1 box Carrot Cake mix, or Spice Cake**
Betty Crocker Super Moist is my favorite!
- **1 can of pumpkin –OR –**
- **1 & ½ cups mashed ripe bananas** (about 4 medium)
- **1 cup grated zucchini** (1 medium)
- **1 cup shredded carrots**
I use the pre-shredded matchstick carrots in the bag.
- **½ cup dried cranberries** (or raisins)

Directions

- Preheat oven to 350°.
- Peel and break bananas into chunks into a medium bowl.
If your bananas are still firm, you can put them in the microwave and cook on high for about 1 minute to soften them.
- Mash the bananas with a potato masher until they are the consistency of chunky baby food.
- Grate (or cut off) the end nub of the zucchini into the trash, then grate the entire zucchini up to the stem (about 1 cup) into the bananas, and stir thoroughly.
- Dump the entire box of dry cake mix into the bowl.
- Stir until thoroughly combined.
- Add 1 cup of shredded carrots and ½ cup of dried cranberries or raisins.
- Stir again until thoroughly combined.

At this point, you will need to decide what you want to make with your delicious batter!

You have several options:

For Mini Muffins...

• Spray muffin tins with non-stick spray, or use a paper towel with butter and wipe all the cups.
• Fill muffin cups heaping to the top with batter.
They will not rise as much as a normal cake batter made with eggs, so be generous!
• Bake for approx. 18-20 minutes at 350°, or until a toothpick comes out clean when poked into the middle of a muffin.
• Remove muffins from the pan and let them cool for a little bit, then dive in and enjoy!!

This will make 24 good size mini muffins.
For regular muffins, bake according to the directions on the box.

For Bundt Cake...

I've also made this as a Bundt Cake and frosted it with Cool Whip Cream Cheese Frosting... deeelicious, and addictive! (Just sayin'. Don't say I didn't warn you!)

• Spray a Bundt pan with non-stick spray, pour all the batter into the pan, and bake according to directions on the box... usually about 40 minutes.

I think this would also be great baked in a mini loaf pan, but I haven't tried it yet. So don't blame me if it doesn't work! Whichever you decide... it's delicious!

$5.00 Family Skillet!

Being a busy mom brings a lot of crazy weeks, and without a plan, it's easy to wind up short-changing my family for dinner! It's really tempting to just hit the drive-thru when life gets hectic, but you can make this ENTIRE meal for your family for the cost of ONE large combo meal! Save the fat and calories, and your cash!

This easy pasta skillet is a deeelicious, inexpensive meal that cooks in no time, and makes more than enough to have left-overs for lunch tomorrow, and the next day! Double it if you want to make enough to freeze for later in the month. (Cook once, eat twice!) Super simple, super fast, super yummy, makes you "Super Mom!" A nice feeling after a week of crazy... Enjoy!!

Ingredients

- **1 box whole grain or wheat pasta**
Rotini, Penne, or Elbow work best.
- **1 pound of lean ground turkey, chicken, or pork**
Chicken or turkey sausage is yummy, too!
- **1 medium white onion- chopped**
- **1 medium zucchini- chopped**
- **2 cans diced Italian tomatoes**
- **2 tablespoons minced garlic**
6 simple ingredients... that's it!!

Directions

- Fill the Pasta Boat 1/2 – 2/3 full with water.

If you don't have a Pasta Boat, buy one... now!! It is the best thing EVER! It cuts your cooking time waaay down! (Check your local thrift stores or discount stores.)

- Microwave water on high for 6 minutes.
- While water is heating, heat a large skillet to med/hi with 2 tablespoons of olive oil.
- Chop one onion and add to skillet.
- Season ground meat and add to skillet.
- Cook until almost done, then chop and add the zucchini... that way they're not squishy!

We have an "NSV Policy" at our house... No Squishy Vegetables!

- When water is done, add one box of pasta to water and stir. The water should cover the pasta.
- Season pasta lightly with salt and stir again.
- Put the Pasta Boat back into the microwave and cook uncovered on high according to directions on package, minus one minute.
- Dump 2 cans of tomatoes (with juice) into the pan and stir.
- Stir in 2 tablespoons of minced garlic.

You can use fresh chopped, or the kind in the jar.

- Cook until meat is done, and turn heat down to low/simmer.

When pasta is done cooking, snap on the locking lid and drain off water... easy peasy! Then quickly rinse in cold water to stop the cooking process and drain again. Don't worry, it will get hot again.

- Dump the pasta into the skillet. Stir and taste test.

At this point I always like to stir in 1 cup of chopped spinach... it looks like a lot, but it cooks down.

To Serve

- Scoop into bowls and enjoy!
- You can also top it with some low fat Parmesan Cheese, if you want... Yummers!

Remember to use your "Fine Chinet" when things are really crazy, and give the "Dish Fairy" a break!   Enjoy!!

Here's a great tip on the spinach!

Buy an extra bag of fresh spinach and throw it in the freezer. When it's completely frozen, take it out and crush it into flakes. Then transfer it to a zip lock freezer bag so you can pull it out and add it to everything! Keep it stocked in the freezer, and you'll always have a great way to discreetly power pack your food with extra color and nutrients!

"Lucky 7 Chili"

This has to be one of my all time favorite recipes! I think I originally got it at a weight loss meeting years ago. It's low fat, high fiber, good lean protein, and... super quick and easy to throw together for dinner in no time! It's also an inexpensive meal that will feed your entire army for pennies on the dollar!

I've named it "Lucky 7 Chili" (777) because it takes 7 cans, preps in under 7 minutes, and costs about $7 for the whole pot, including leftovers! You will definitely "hit the jackpot" with this meal! Enjoy!

Ingredients

- 2 cans dark red kidney beans
- 1 can black beans
- 1 can white beans
- 1 can sweet corn
- 1 can diced Mexican (or Italian) tomatoes
- 1 can Mexican stewed tomatoes
- 1 white onion- chopped
- 1 package of powdered taco seasoning

For the meat...
- You can use an entire 20 oz. package of LEAN ground turkey, ground pork, or ground beef.
However... Remember to "Cook once, eat twice!"

Buy 1- 20 oz. package of lean ground meat and cook it all. Then use 1/2 of the meat for the chili. Put the other 1/2 in the fridge and use it for spaghetti sauce, our $5.00 Skillet, or tacos later in the week! Done, and done! ☺

If you want Southwest Chicken Chili, you can add cut up cooked chicken breast, about 1 & 1/2 – 2 cups, depending on how much meat you like. You can also use 1 can of chunk chicken if you're really short on time!

Directions for Stovetop

• Add 1 tablespoon of olive oil into the bottom of a medium size stockpot. Heat on med/hi and wait for the pot to get hot.
• Add one chopped onion and all the ground meat into the bottom of the skillet.
• Season with season salt and pepper.
• Cook until done... about 4-5 minutes.
• Add 1 tablespoon of minced garlic into meat mixture and stir.
If you are splitting the meat, scoop out ½ for later.
• Drain all the beans and the corn.
• Do NOT drain tomatoes. The juice adds great flavor to your chili!
• Dump the kidney beans, black beans, white beans, corn, and tomatoes into the pot. Stir thoroughly.
• Depending on your salt intake, sprinkle the taco seasoning accordingly. I have found that it doesn't need a lot of extra seasoning. Start with about 1/2 a package and taste to see if you like it. If not, add more. It will get stronger as it cooks.
• Stir and cover.

• Cook on low heat for 1-2 hours, depending on how "sludgy" you like your chili. The longer it goes, the more it breaks down. Make sure to stir it occasionally.
Buy your favorite easy cornbread mix to make just before dinner and enjoy!

Crock Pot Directions

• Follow the same steps for cooking your meat and draining the beans.

• Dump the onions, all the cans, and the meat into a medium size Crock Pot and stir.

• Add seasoning, and stir again.

• Cover and cook on low for 4 hours, or on high for 2 hours.

• Serve with cornbread and enjoy!!

Pork Veggie Burger Sliders

I love a good burger! I used to eat burgers a whole lot more than I do now. So now when I do have one, I want a really good one, but I try to look for a lower fat version!

I always LOVE to find ways to add veggies to our meals, so this burger starts with sautéed onions, mushrooms, and spinach. Then I add those veggies into my meat to make veggie burger patties. I make them smaller so they'll cook faster (of course!)... then I brown them in a skillet, and serve them with a side salad and BBQ Black Beans! Total cost for 8 sliders and all the extras? Less than ONE large burger combo meal at the drive-thru! Now that's a bargain!!

Ingredients

- **1/2 pound lean ground pork** (or turkey)
- **1 onion minced**
- **1 good size (3-4 inch) Portobello mushroom**
Or 6 smaller white or brown mushrooms
- **1/2 cup crushed frozen spinach flakes**
I always freeze an additional fresh bag to use later!
- **Hotdog buns** (No, that is not a type-o!)
- **Season with seasoned salt and garlic pepper,**
and other seasonings.
- Sometimes I will cut a light cheese stick into tiny pieces and mixed it in to make "cheeseburgers"!
Yummers!

Directions

- Heat a nonstick skillet to med/hi with 2 tbls. of Olive oil.
- Chop onion and add to hot pan.
- Chop mushroom(s) and add to pan.
- Season, and sauté for 2-3 minutes.
- Add 1/2 cup frozen, chopped spinach and cook for another 2 minutes.
- Remove pan from heat.
- In separate bowl, combine a 1/2 pound (or 1/2 a package) of lean, ground meat.
- Season with salt, pepper, and garlic. Stir until combined.
- Add all the veggie mixture into the raw meat and stir until thoroughly combined.
- Reheat your skillet to med/hi heat with another 1 tablespoon of Olive oil.
- Shape burger mix into small patties, approx. 2 & 1/2 inches around.
(Remember when you are using lean meat, it will not shrink as much as a high fat beef burger!)
- Brown burgers on both sides and cook through.
- Cut hog dog buns in half.
- Place one burger on each bun.

They're ya go... 2 for the price of 1! You're welcome! ☺

BBQ Black Beans

When it starts heatin' up on the outside, the last thing I want to do is heat up my house on the inside! So, I avoid using my oven as often as possible once it's officially Summer.

With all the backyard chillin' and grillin' going on, you need a great side dish that will stand up to all that great BBQ! These BBQ Black Beans have become my favorite side dish when we grill! I add extra onion and garlic (Yummers!), and I do them in the microwave in just minutes... super simple, and I get to keep the heat outside!

Not only are they deeelicious, but they also have approximately 1 gram of fat, 7 grams of fiber, and 7 grams of protein in just a ½- cup! And, with black beans coming in under a buck a can... that's a super side dish that just makes CENTS! Enjoy!

This recipe only makes about 4 small servings, so I would definitely double it if you want to have more for guests!

Ingredients

- 1 can low sodium black beans
- 1 medium white onion
- 1 tbls. minced garlic
- ¼-cup honey bbq sauce
My favorite is Kraft Thick 'n Spicy Honey!
- 1 tablespoon of honey or packed brown sugar

Directions

- Dice one onion into very small pieces.
- Place onions in the bottom of a wide, shallow microwave-safe bowl and spread out on the bottom... or you could brown them in a skillet.
- Add one tablespoon minced garlic and about 1 teaspoon of water. Stir to combine.
- Lightly season onions with salt.
- Microwave on high for about 3 minutes, or until onions are soft.
- Open the can of black beans and drain.
- Pull the bowl out of the microwave and stir.
- Dump the beans into the bowl and stir.
- Mash some of the beans until they get a little 'sludgy'. *We don't want them to look like refried beans, but we do want them to stick together a bit!*
- Stir it all up again.
- Put the beans into the microwave and cook, uncovered, on high for 3 minutes.
- When the time is done, pull them out and add 1/4 cup of HONEY BBQ sauce. Stir until combined.
- Add 1 tablespoon of packed brown sugar, or honey, and stir again!
- Put the beans back in the microwave and cook on medium/high (70%ish power) for another 3 minutes.
- BE CAREFUL... the dish will be VERY HOT!!
- *Serve immediately; reheat before serving later.*

Garlic Dill Potatoes

We all need a good 'go to' side dish that's quick and easy to make, and just as deeelicious to eat! This is one of my favorite ways to fix a low fat potato side dish that will compliment any meal! It works great with steak, chicken, pork, or fish... whatever you wish!

When Spring and Summer come around, these will be especially delicious along side all that great grillin' in the backyard... Enjoy!

Ingredients

- **1 small bag (about 18-20) of small colored potatoes, about 2 inches around**
Or just the red ones work great!
- **2 tablespoons of Garlic Butter**
I LOVE "I Can't Believe it's Not Butter". Lower fat!
- **Dry dill flakes**
- **Garlic salt & pepper**
- **Fresh garlic – optional**

Directions

- Wash the potatoes thoroughly to remove dirt.
- Cut potatoes into quarters, or smaller, and place them into a microwave safe bowl.
- If you want to use fresh garlic, smash, peel, and dice it now, and stir it into the potatoes.
- Season with season salt, garlic salt, and pepper, and toss the potatoes to get them all covered with the seasoning. *Remember, a little seasoning goes a looong way... you can always add later, but you can't take it back!*

- Add a splash of water in the bottom of the bowl to keep the potatoes moist when they cook.
- Stir, and cook on high for 6 minutes.
- Check to see if they are done. If not, add extra minutes accordingly.
You want them to be tender enough to poke them with a fork, but still firm enough to hold together.
- When the potatoes are finished cooking, season lightly with additional garlic salt, if needed.
- Add 2 tablespoons of Garlic Butter to the entire bowl of warm potatoes and toss to coat.
- When potatoes are coated, generously sprinkle dry dill over the potatoes and stir. Repeat and stir again until they look and taste the way you want.

Serve warm for best flavor, and prepare to have your taste buds dance with joy!!

(I love them with Dill Salmon!)

Heirloom Tomato Salad

Every year our family heads toward the CA coast for one last "hurrah" before school begins, and it's always one of my favorite weeks of the year!

One year we found a fresh Farmer's Market down on the main street of the nearby town of Pescadero. Oh my goodness! Huge, fresh, heirloom tomatoes, ginormous peaches and nectarines, and varieties of crossbred fruit in colors and flavors that I'd never seen before! SO incredibly delicious!

They had samples of everything out for tasting, so, of course, we did! (It would just be rude not to, right?!) One of the samples was a fresh tomato salad. We loved it so much that we went to the little country market across the street, bought the extra ingredients, and went back to our campsite to make it that night for dinner! I loved it so much, I just had to share it with you... you're welcome!

I know that Heirloom tomatoes can be pricey, but considering the money you're saving every time you "ditch the drive-thru", it's worth a splurge just for the flavor and color! Serve it in place of heavy potato salad with a turkey burger for a change, or along side our Chicken Tortilla Soup recipe... SO deeelicious and SO good for you! Enjoy!

Ingredients

- **3 large heirloom tomatoes- 1 red, 1 orange, 1 yellow**
- **Low fat Feta cheese**
- **Cilantro**
- **1 cucumber**
- **Olive oil**
- **Salt and pepper, to taste**

Directions

- Cut the tomatoes into chunks, about 1-inch pieces.
- Peel the cucumber and dice into smaller pieces.
- Rough chop some cilantro and add to the salad.
Depending on how much you like Cilantro, look at the color balance and add more if you think it needs it!
- Drizzle the salad with olive oil, and gently mix until combined.
- Add the crumbled Feta cheese, again to taste.
If you like it salty, add a little more... but don't let it overpower the tomatoes!
- Stir again, and season with salt and pepper to taste.
- Serve slightly chilled for best flavor, and enjoy!!

I do recommend only making as much as you think you'll eat... it keeps for maybe a day in the fridge, but tends to get soggy. Since you can throw it together so quickly, it's always better to make it fresh! Yummers!

Strawberry Spinach Salad

As I continue to meet more vegetarians, I am always interested in finding delicious options that will satisfy not only their dietary guidelines, but their taste buds, as well! I'm a self-declared, "meat-a-tarian"! (That's what I call a person who loves veggies, but likes meat too much to give it up!) However, I love finding delicious, all-veggie meal options!

This is, by far, one of my very favorite, most delicious, scrumptious, beautiful, nutrient rich, power-packed salads of all time! Are you hungry yet?! Fresh spinach, fresh strawberries, and a delicious low fat Raspberry Vinaigrette topped with all the extra goodies make this as yummy as a 'dessert' salad! So delicious, so nutritious, and all the ingredients will be in season in the coming months! Deeelicious!

Ingredients

- 1 bag Fresh Express Spinach
- 1 container fresh strawberries
- 1/2 cup slivered raw almonds
- 1/2 cup grated (matchstick) carrots
- 1 large avocado
- Low fat small croutons
- LITE Raspberry Vinaigrette Salad Dressing

Directions

- Wash and slice strawberries for the salad.
- Layer each item onto individual plates...
    - 2 large handfuls of spinach
    - 3 or 4 sliced strawberries
    - 1 handful of matchstick carrots
    - 1 handful slivered raw almonds
    - 1/4 of 1 large chopped avocado
- Top with 1 tablespoon LITE Raspberry Vinaigrette, and add croutons and real bacon bit pieces, if desired!

Serve immediately and enjoy!!

Chinese Chicken Salad

I once overheard some ladies talking about their version of Chinese Chicken Salad, and I really should have given them my recipe instead! They were talking about marinating the chicken... and cooking the chicken... who wants to be doing that when we could be swimming or enjoying the outdoors on our day off?!

My recipe is super quick and easy, and it is goodness in a bowl! Most Chinese Chicken Salads are chocked FULL of fat and calories, but, of course, NOT our "Ditch the Drive-Thru!" version. This low fat version will make you wonder why you've ever made it any other way. And when people tell you that they just can't believe you went to 'all the trouble' to make such an amazing salad for their gathering, just smile and nod, take a bite, and chew on your delicious salad secret! We won't tell... enjoy!

Ingredients

- 1 bag angel hair coleslaw
- 1/2 bag tri-color coleslaw
- 1 (15oz.) can mandarin oranges (cut into halves)
- 1 (12.5oz.) can chunk chicken
- 1cup slivered almonds (or a 4 oz. bag)
- 1/2 cup LOW FAT (light) Asian dressing

Directions

Dump 'n Dine! ☺

What?!
You were expecting something more difficult? HA!

Ok, so here's the step-by-step for the rest of you...
• Open both bags of cabbage. Dump all of the angel hair and 1/2 of the tri-color cabbage into a LARGE bowl. You need room to mix it up!
• Open the can of chicken and drain. Shred it a little in the can, and then dump into the bowl and stir.
• Open oranges and drain off juice.
• Cut oranges into halves, dump into bowl, and stir.
• Add ½-cup of LITE Asian Salad Dressing on top of the salad and stir until thoroughly mixed.
Taste to make sure that the dressing is the proper amount for your salad. If it needs more, add a little at a time until it it's just right. It's really strong and you don't need a lot!
• If you are going to serve your salad immediately, add ¾-cup slivered almonds into the salad and stir until combined. Garnish each salad with the ¼-cup of remaining almonds when you serve it!
Otherwise, hold the almonds out and wait to stir them in right before you serve it later.

** You can also top it with instant Ramen Noodles. Add them on top right before you serve it.
If you mix them into the salad they get mushy! They also add more empty calories, so that's why I've gone with the almonds!

• Scoop onto plates and enjoy!

Sweet 'n Sour Pork

When we have an opportunity to eat out as a family, we will usually choose Chinese food. We LOVE Chinese Food! It's SO deeelicious, but SO full of fat and calories!! My husband often orders Sweet 'n Sour Pork, which is SO good, but not something I eat often, because of all the calories!

So, in true "Ditch the Drive-Thru!" fashion, I needed to find my own make-at-home version that my hubby would love! I've found that my version of low fat Sweet 'n Sour Pork satisfies my taste buds (and his!) just fine without all the extra calories.

No coating, no deep-frying... just yummy Sweet 'n Sour Pork in no time at all, and it's much less expensive than taking the whole family out for dinner! Enjoy!

Ingredients

- **3 cups (approx.) of 1 inch cubed pork**
- **1 large white onion, chopped**
- **1 large yellow pepper**
- **1 large green pepper**
- **1 large red pepper**
- **1 can pineapple chunks in juice**
- **1/2-cup matchstick carrots**
- **1 bottle of your favorite sweet 'n sour sauce**
- **1 bag steamer brown rice**
- **1 bag steamer fried rice**

I have used Barley, as well... very yummy!

Directions

- Heat a large skillet to med/hi heat with 3 tablespoons of Olive oil.
- Put one bag of brown rice into the microwave, and cook on high according to the package.
- Season pork with seasoned salt and pepper.
- Chop onion and peppers into 1 inch pieces.
- When pan is hot, put pork into pan.
Watch out, it may spatter!
- Brown pork quickly, flipping pieces to lightly brown the meat on all sides.
- When the first bag of rice is done, pull it out, and put fried rice bag into microwave. Again, cook according to directions on package.
- As soon as the pork is slightly browned, add onion and peppers.
- Stir, and continue to cook for 3-4 more minutes.
- Open and drain the can of pineapple chunks.
- Dump the pineapple into pan.
- Add 1/2-cup matchstick carrots for extra color, and stir again.
- Dump the entire bottle of Sweet 'n Sour Sauce into the pan, and stir.
- Turn heat down to low and cover until ready to serve.
- Take second bag of rice out of the microwave.
- Combine brown rice and fried rice together in a bowl and stir until mixed.

To serve...
- Scoop rice onto plates, and top with Sweet 'n Sour Pork. Give yourself a big "WooHoo" for another opportunity to *"Ditch the Drive-Thru!"*

"Chow-Ra-Mein!"

It's no secret that I LOVE Chinese food! If I have a choice to eat out, it will usually be a toss up between Chinese or Sushi, depending on whether I'm in the mood for hot or cold... and what I want to spend!

I've never been a huge fan of Ramen noodles, simply because they are _super_ high in sodium and don't have a whole lot of nutritional value. However, they are very inexpensive and kids just seem to love them! Soooo, I figured there must be SOME way to add some nutritional value, and get my Chinese food fix at the same time!

I started thinking about a quick and easy way to make Chow mein, and I've got it! My "Chow-Ra-Mein" is a super easy, low fat, much less expensive version of traditional Chinese Chow mein, and a whole lot less work! Once you get it down, you'll be done in about 7 minutes... faster than a restaurant, that's for sure!

I demonstrate how to make this dish when I'm out with Sacramento Food Bank and Family Services, and it's been a HUGE hit! Their clients LOVE it!

Using Oriental Ramen Noodles that you can find for about 20¢ a package, this is a great way to get those veggies into your kids, and add some good, lean protein as well. (Not to mention, saving another expensive trip to eat out at a restaurant!)

Serve this with some chicken and steamed broccoli, or our Chinese Chicken Salad, and you'll have a great meal that your family will love for a fraction of the cost! Enjoy!

Ingredients

- **2 packages of Oriental Flavor Ramen Noodles**
- **2 cups of water**
- **1 Oriental flavor packet**
- **2 stalks of celery**
- **1/2 head of green cabbage**
- **1 medium white onion**
- **1 handful of shredded carrots**

I buy the pre-shredded bag at the 99¢ Store!

- **1 cup of frozen sweet peas** (optional)

If you want to add meat, here are some options:

- **1 package of lean, cooked chicken strips**

You can also use a can of chunk chicken, or shredded lean pork.

- **If you're a vegetarian, try cubed firm tofu instead!**

Directions

- Heat a large skillet to med/hi heat with 2 tablespoons of Olive oil.
- Remove Ramen Noodles from the package.
- Split the bricks open in half and place in a wide, shallow, microwave dish.
- Add 2 cups of water in the bottom, and sprinkle 1/2 of 1 package of seasoning over the noodles and into the water.
- Cook on high for 3 minutes in the microwave.
- Slice each end off the onion. Cut in half, and then slice into thin strips. Add the onions into the hot skillet and get cooking!
- Wash and slice the celery thinly on the diagonal, and set aside.
- Rinse and cut the cabbage into quarters, then cut into strips.
- Add the celery and cabbage into pan. Stir to combine, and continue cooking.

- Season the veggies with a little salt and pepper and 'stir fry' for about 3 minutes.
(I love Lawry's Seasoned Salt and Garlic Pepper!)
- Add 1 cup of shredded carrots (a generous handful) and stir.
- Add 1 cup of peas, and the chicken strips if you're adding meat.
- Sprinkle the rest of the seasoning packet over the veggies and stir. Continue cooking until hot.
- When noodles are done, dump the noodles and broth into the pan. Some of the liquid will cook down, but still keep it moist.
- Stir to combine.
- Season the entire pan with the other 1/2 package of oriental seasoning, and stir again. (You could add a little low sodium soy sauce if you want, but you probably won't need it!)
- Serve hot and enjoy!

Pan-Seared Salmon

Broccoli & Sweet Potatoes

I LOVE salmon, but I have to admit that it can be somewhat expensive for as often as I'd like to eat it. If you are looking for a cheaper alternative, try the frozen bags with vacuum packed pieces. (I buy a bag of 4 nice pieces of frozen salmon at my low price grocery store for around $5.00.)

Thaw them in the microwave if you're short on time and then throw them into a hot skillet for a couple of minutes. Throw back those scrawny, little fish sticks, and catch this delicious fish instead... you'll make a splash with dinner in no time!

Remember, watch out for the sauce! Sauces can easily add up to 10+ extra grams of fat to your healthy, low fat meal! Look for a low fat tarter sauce, if you must have it, and save the extra fat and calories for dessert! Yummers!

Ingredients

- 4 pieces of salmon
- 4 sweet potatoes (yams)
- 2 crowns fresh broccoli
- Butter for potatoes

Directions

- Thaw salmon overnight in fridge -OR-
- Place individually frozen pieces in bags in the microwave.
- Cook on high for 1 minute, check for defrosting, add 1 minute more if necessary.
- Heat a large skillet to med/hi with 2 tbls. Olive oil.
- Pierce 4 medium sized sweet potatoes several times through and put in microwave.
- Cook potatoes on high for 5 minutes.

While potatoes are cooking...
- Season salmon with salt and pepper.
I always use a season salt and garlic pepper.
- Place salmon, top side down, into hot skillet... cook for about 2 minutes, until browned.

While salmon is cooking...
- Wash and cut broccoli into small/med florets.
- Lightly season broccoli florets with salt and pepper. *(See above!)*
- Flip salmon over and add broccoli into pan around the salmon.
- Cook for about 2 minutes.
- Turn off heat and cover. Move pan off heat. Let it sit for about another 2 minutes.
- Check potatoes to make sure they are soft. If not done, cook on high again about 1 – 1 & 1/2 minutes.
- Serve 1 piece of salmon, 1 sweet potato, and a generous portion of broccoli onto plates.

- Check the clock and notice that it only took you about 12 minutes to make this FAAABULOUS dinner, and enjoy!

Also try a Salmon Veggie Rice Bowl...

It's super quick, super healthy, and MUCH less expensive than the drive-thru!

• Prepare the salmon the same way.

While the fish is cooking...

• Open and combine 1 bag steamer brown rice and 1 bag steamer mixed veggies into microwave safe bowl, stir to mix.
• Heat on high for 4 minutes, or until hot, stirring 1/2 way through.
• Scoop veggie rice into bowls and top with salmon when it's finished... deeelicious!

Tilapia Fish Tacos

Our local taco shop makes the BEST Crispy Fish Tacos! They taste SO good, but are SO bad on the fat... one drive-thru version has 17 grams in just one! (And let's be honest, who really eats just one? C'mon.)

My goal is always to find ways to recreate my yummy drive-thru favorites at home for much less fat and calories, and these fish tacos do not disappoint! They're deeelicious!

Ingredients

- **Small fajita size tortillas**
- **4 pieces of Tilapia fillets**
I buy the bag with individually frozen pieces.
- **1 bag angel hair coleslaw**
- Pico de Gallo
You can find it in the produce department.
- **Avocado** (I use 1 small avocado for 4 tacos.)

To garnish~
You can add light sour cream, low fat finely shredded cheese, and a squirt of lime, if you want!

Directions

- If Tilapia is frozen, defrost pieces in the microwave before cooking.
- Heat a large, non-stick skillet to medium/hi heat with 2 tbls. Olive oil.
- Season Tilapia fillets

Try a little season salt and some garlic pepper. Yum!

- Place fish in pan and cook until done on the bottom.

Flip fish and cook the other side.

- While fish is cooking, heat tortillas on each side in a separate non-stick skillet on medium and pile on a plate.
- When fish is cooked, split Tilapia pieces down the middle so you get 2 pieces of fish from each fillet.
- Turn off heat and remove pan from burner.

To assemble:
- Start with 1 tortilla, add 1 piece of Tilapia, shredded cabbage, Pico de Gallo, and freshly chopped avocado.
- Top with a little light sour cream, some low fat finely shredded cheese, and a squirt of lime juice.
- Repeat and make 2 fish tacos per person. Make more or less depending on your family. Enjoy!!

6 Can - Chicken Tortilla Soup

I LOVE Chicken Tortilla Soup! It actually comes in fairly low on the calorie count at one well-known Mexican restaurant drive-thru, but sometimes I want to make it at home, too! This recipe is so quick and easy, and so deeelicious! Enjoy!

(Original recipe from All Recipes.com makes approx. 6 servings.)

Ingredients

- **2 (14.5 ounce) cans chicken broth** (or 32 oz. box)
- **1 (10 ounce) can chunk chicken** (or 1 cup chopped chicken)
- **1 (15 ounce) can black beans**
- **1 (15 ounce) can sweet whole kernel corn, drained**
- **1 (10 ounce) can diced tomatoes with green chilies,** drained
Use either mild or spicy, depending on your taste buds!
- **Fresh Cilantro for garnish-** chopped
- **1 large avocado- chopped**
- **Low fat finely shredded cheese**
Mexican or Colby/Jack are best!
You can also use low fat crumbled feta cheese!
- **1 package tri-color tortilla strips**
Or low(er) fat tortilla chips- crushed

Directions

- Dump chicken broth into a large pot.
- Drain all cans and add into the broth.
- I also like to add about an 1/8-ish (?) of a cup of chopped cilantro!
  (It adds great flavor and color!)
- Stir until combined.
- Heat until hot... done and done!

To Serve

Ladle soup into bowls and top with a scoop of chopped avocado, a small amount of shredded cheese or Feta, tortilla strips, and fresh cilantro. Deeelicious!

Chicken Pot Pie Soup

I am convinced that you can throw almost anything into a skillet, brown it up, pour in some sauce or chicken broth, and call it dinner! In this case, it turned into creamy soup... and reeeeaally delicious, creamy soup, I might add!

Chicken Pot Pie has a ridiculous amount of fat and calories... especially if you order it in a drive-thru or at a restaurant! So the next time you're in the mood for 'comfort food', try this low fat alternative instead! It will warm your heart _and_ your tummy! Enjoy!

Ingredients

- **10 chicken tenderloin pieces**
- **1 onion**
- **1 cup of chopped broccoli florets** (fresh or frozen)
- **1/2 package of mixed vegetables**
- **1 can low fat Cream of Chicken soup**
- **1/2 can low fat milk** (about 1 cup)

Directions

- Heat a non-stick skillet to med/hi with 1 tablespoon of Olive oil.
- Add chicken tenderloin pieces to pan.

You can substitute a can of chunk chicken for this, if you don't have tenderloins on hand.

- Cook chicken 'til almost done, and break apart into smaller, bite-size pieces.
- Chop and add one onion into pan.
- Add the rest of the veggies into the pan and season.

I use a Seasoned Salt, Garlic Salt, and Garlic Pepper!

- Sauté veggies until tender, but firm.
- Add one can low fat Cream of Chicken Soup.
- Add one can of water and 1/2 can of low fat milk.
- Stir all the ingredients until thoroughly combined.
- Turn the heat down to simmer and let the soup cook for a few minutes until everything is hot.

Serve warm with some hot, low(er) fat biscuits!
Don't forget to pop them into the oven when you start your soup so they'll be done and ready to serve at the same time!

This recipe makes 4 generous bowls! Enjoy!

Chicken Pot Pie

This recipe is SO fast and delicious... and waaaaay less calories and fat than traditional potpie! It definitely hits the spot when you're in the mood for some good old-fashioned "comfort food"! Keep extra frozen veggies on hand, and a couple of extra cans of soup and chicken in your pantry so you can "Ditch the Drive-Thru!"

You can throw this dinner together in NO time and your family will love it! Once again, it's Campbell's Soup to the rescue!

Ingredients

- 1 can low fat Cream of Chicken Soup
- 1/2 can low fat milk
- 1 package frozen mixed veggies

Peas, carrots, corn, and green beans work best.

- 1 – 12oz can of chunk chicken
- 1 package refrigerator biscuits -OR-
- 1 package refrigerator crescent rolls

Directions

- Dump veggies into a microwave <u>and</u> oven safe dish.
A 9 x 9 inch, or a 9-inch pie dish work great!
- Drain chicken and add into veggies... stir, and season with seasoned salt and pepper if desired.
- Add 1 can low fat Cream of Chicken Soup with 1/2 a can of low fat milk... stir again until combined.
- Cook in the microwave on high for 10 minutes.

While this is cooking, get out your biscuits.
If you are using Biscuits...
- Cut each one into quarters and place all over the top, covering the filling.
- Bake according to biscuit directions on package... usually another 10 minutes in the oven at 350° does the trick!

If you are using Crescent Rolls...
- Unroll each piece and lay out on top of the filling, covering as much as possible.
- Again, bake according to directions on the package... about the same amount of time.

NOTE- this recipe works great with either kind of dough... it just depends on what mood you're in.
If you want a "Chicken 'n Dumplings" style dish, then use quartered biscuits. If you want more of a traditional pot pie crust, use the Crescent Rolls. Either one is delicious, but using biscuits does make it lower in fat.

- Let stand 5 minutes before serving, but serve hot!

Easy Chicken Tortilla Casserole

This recipe is so easy and so delicious, and I haven't really ever found anything else like it. It's ooey, gooey, and full of yummy for your tummy! (It's my Mom's specialty and I love it!) It also makes a great big '9 x 13' casserole with low cost, low fat ingredients... and gives you enough leftovers for another meal!

Serve it up with a nice side salad, and you have a delicious (mostly nutritious) meal! Feed your whole family for a few dollars, and then take a serving with you to work for lunch the next day for more scrumptious savings! Enjoy!

Ingredients

- **1 chicken cooked and cubed**
You can buy a cooked chicken in the deli, or use 2 cans of chunk chicken if you don't want the extra work!
Precooked chicken strips also work great, but chop them into smaller pieces.
- **2 cans low fat Cream of Chicken Soup**
- **1-cup light sour cream**
- **1 small can mild green chilies**
- **1/2 pound low fat Jack cheese**
(You can also use Colby Jack or Mexican Fiesta!)
- **8 'lower fat' flour tortillas- read the labels!**

Directions

- Tear or cut tortillas into 3 inch pieces, and set aside.
This is a great way to get the kids involved!
- Spray a 9×13 inch pan with non-stick cooking spray.
- Divide ingredients evenly and spread over pan in the following order:
  Tortillas, Cream of Chicken Soup, Sour Cream, Green Chilies, Chicken...
- Repeat these steps again.
- Finish with remaining tortillas, and cover the top with cheese.

** *In the interest of 'full disclosure', my Mom says that she just tears up the tortillas, mixes it all together in a bowl, and throws it into the pan. I think that's a new development because I distinctly remember standing and layering all the ingredients into the pan! I like the layers, but her new way would definitely be faster!* ☺

- Bake at 350° for 45 minutes.

- Let stand 5 minutes before serving, but serve hot.
- Makes approximately 8 nice size servings, or 12 smaller portions.

Serve it with a delicious, colorful salad on the side, and you have a wonderful meal that is sure to please the whole family!

Tuna Noodle Casserole

Do you remember Tuna Noodle Casserole from when you were a kid? My Mom didn't make it a lot, but I know it's something I liked because it was creamy and had peas in it! (I love sweet peas!)

The 'traditional' version of this can be pretty time consuming, and it is loaded with fat and calories! I've seen everything from 20 minutes to one hour for prep and cook, and high calorie ingredients like evaporated milk, 3 cups of cheese, "cooking crèmes", and even potato chips!

Try this instead...

This is my quick and easy version of Tuna Noodle Casserole... on the table in less than 15 minutes! It makes enough to have leftovers for lunch the next day, and all for around just $5.00 for the whole dish! It's just another a great way to feed your family, and save your cash and calories.

Ingredients

- **1 box of Garden Veggie Rotini noodles**
I like the way the sauce gets stuck in the spirals and the colors make it look pretty! You can use medium shells, or traditional egg noodles, as well.
- **1 jar of Ragu LIGHT Parmesan Alfredo Sauce**
(My "Pasta Voila" Sauce!)
- **1 can of chunk light tuna in water**
- **1 cup of sweet frozen peas**
- **Parmesan Cheese for topping**

Directions

- Fill Pasta Boat 1/2 full with water and cook on high in the microwave for 6 minutes.
- While water is heating, measure 1 cup of sweet peas into a small bowl and set aside to defrost.
- When water is hot, dump the box of pasta into water. Season with salt, add a little olive oil, and stir.
- Cook on high, uncovered, according to directions on box, minus one minute. (Usually about 7-9 minutes)
- Prepare a side salad while the noodles are cooking. *Pre-bagged salads are great way to save time!*
- When noodles are finished, add 1 cup of peas into the water and stir BEFORE draining! This gets your peas hot without cooking them.
- Snap on the Pasta Boat strainer lid. Lock the lid and drain off water, leaving about ¼ cup in the bottom.
- Open and drain tuna, and add tuna into pasta.
- Open Parmesan Alfredo Sauce, shout "Voilaaah!", and dump into the Pasta Boat.
- Stir all the ingredients until everything is well mixed.
Serve immediately with a side salad. Enjoy!

Chocolate Covered

Strawberry Sundaes!

I have always LOVED the 4th of July! I love spending the day with my family, I love BBQ, I love corn on the cob, I love sparklers when it's dark, and I LOVE fireworks that light up the sky! Most of all, I love this special day to be reminded of why America is still the greatest country on earth!

One of our family traditions has become Chocolate Covered Strawberry Sundaes while we wait for fireworks to start! Mmm, mmmm! This is SO delicious I just HAD to share it with you!

I LOVE chocolate covered strawberries, and this sundae is the closest I've found without all the melting and dipping work. I slice the strawberries and put them into a container before we leave, and then we pack our ice cream in ice in an ice chest. As soon as we find our spot, we set up and dish out dessert!

This is a great sundae to serve to guests after a backyard BBQ, too! It's super quick because your strawberries can be sliced ahead, and it has great "wow factor", which is always a bonus... Enjoy!!

Ingredients

- **1 container of fresh strawberries**
Buy a larger one if you're serving more people!
- **1 half gallon of low(er) fat vanilla ice cream**
My favorite is Dreyer's Slow Churned... it's deeelicious!
- **1 bottle Chocolate Fudge Magic Shell**
- **1 can low fat spray whipped cream**
- **Optional - chocolate fudge brownies**

Directions

- Wash and thinly slice strawberries into a bowl.
- Sprinkle with sugar and squish gently 3 or 4 times while stirring to get the juices to start coming out of the berries; set aside.
- If you are using a brownie on the bottom, place one (2×2-ish inch) brownie in the bottom of a bowl.
- Add a good scoop of low fat vanilla, or vanilla with chocolate marble, ice cream on top of the brownie.
- Scoop a nice serving of strawberries onto the ice cream and around the bottom of the bowl.
- Pour Magic Shell over the ice cream and the berries (not too thick) and let it harden. Don't worry... it only takes about a minute!
- Finish with whip cream and one berry on top!

I always say, "Half of food is the presentation!"

Serve your family their bowl of deeelicious-ness, and get ready to enjoy your evening of lots of "oooh's" and "aaaah's"! ... and I'm not just talking about the fireworks! Enjoy!

"Mug Cakes"

I have found my new favorite dessert! These are SO simple...
and so deeelicious! LOW FAT, and done in *less than
1 minute*! Does it get any better? I think not!!

The concept is simple:

- **1 tablespoon of white Angel Food Cake mix**
- **2 tablespoons of your favorite flavored cake mix**
- **2 tablespoons water**

- Mix all ingredients in a coffee mug and whip until frothy.
- Cook on high in the microwave for 40 seconds.
- Top it with a scoop of low fat ice cream, or flip it over onto
a plate and decorate with your favorite toppings! The
possibilities are endless... Enjoy!

*Try a "Make-Your-Own-Mug-Cake-Bar" for a party, with several
flavor combinations for your guests.
 If you need some more inspiration, you can download the
recipes from our website:*

www.ditchthedrive-thru.com

You can also find additional ideas and more great recipes
on our Facebook Page at facebook.com/ditchthedrivethru.

"Ditch the Drive-Thru!"
· Nutrition Education for a Future Generation ·

Tips for Family Dinnertime!

Congratulations on your quest to

"Ditch the Drive-Thru!".

If you haven't had a family dinner

together in a while, or ever,

here are some tips to help you establish

your new family "table time".

You may want to review these with your family
so everyone knows the expectations!

#1 – NO CELL PHONES... *Period!*

ALL electronic devices are banned! Put them on SILENT or turn them off! Some families use a basket and everyone deposits their phones until dinner is done! Here's the thing: unless you are in the middle of a family emergency (as in, someone's in the hospital!) and you need to take a phone call, it can wait!! This means texting, too! Tell your BFF that U will call her L8R and LOL all NITE! Dinnertime is FAMILY time, and time to reconnect. It's "Face Time" with each other, NOT with your iPhone!

It makes me SO angry when I see a family out to eat in a nice restaurant with everyone buried in their cell phone screens or tablets, completely ignoring the people they're with at the table!! It's even worse when it happens at home! I mean it! No work, no friends, no social media, no checking emails, no texting, or anything else during the time that you are having dinner together! Whatever it is can wait for the short half hour that you are actually sitting down at the dinner table together! Be PRESENT... *be with your family!*

#2 – Expect your children to be "squirrely"!

If your children are not used to sitting down and behaving during dinner, you CANNOT expect them to be little angels! They are going to be restless and squirrely! You need to be prepared to remind them of good table manners, and help them be successful. It will take practice, and patience! Keep the 'big picture' in mind... remember, you are helping your family "change the nutritional environment of your home"!

#3 – Have a plan for "time fillers".

There are some really fun, simple, silly games that you can play with your family! My husband will occasionally play "Would You Rather?" with our kids while I'm getting the last items on the table.

This is a 'game of preference' so keep in mind that there are no "wrong" answers, and everyone gets to share their opinion without being interrupted! I even found this game at a thrift store for a few dollars, so now we have the question cards on the table to refer to, instead of making them up!

Here are a few questions to get you started:

Ask your kids, *"Would you rather..."*

... be named after a car, or be named after produce? (vegetables and fruit)

... be stuck on the moon, or stuck at the bottom of the ocean?

... spend a day in the Sahara Desert, or a day in the North Pole?

... be an elephant, or be a mouse?

... have knee length hair, or have a 1 foot tall Mohawk?

... be stuck in traffic for 4 hours, or be stranded in the mountains?

... be trapped in an aquarium with a Great White Shark, or walk across a floor filled with spiders?

#4 – Teach your children good table manners!

Manners are a lost art in our society! No one knows how to sit at the table, or even use a knife and fork properly anymore! We reach across the table, we pick up our plates, we shovel our food in, we chew with our mouths open, and we are done eating almost as soon as the food hits the table! It's atrocious!! It's time for us to teach our children, and also remind ourselves, how to use good table manners! Here are a few tips:

1. Pull the chair up to the table and sit up straight.

2. Use a fork, knife, and napkin! Unless you are eating 'finger food', use the utensils properly!

3. Ask for things to be passed, instead of reaching across the table!

4. **Always say**, "Excuse me", "Please", and "Thank you".

5. Slow down when you are eating!

   Teach your children to chew each bite 20 times before swallowing. It may seem like a lot, but it helps to keep those mouths closed when chewing, and it helps with digestion. It takes 20 minutes for your stomach to tell your brain it's full!

6. Ask to be excused from the table when the meal is done.

   We say, "Thank you for my dinner, may I please be excused?"

   Please note... just because someone is done in 5 minutes, doesn't mean they need to be excused. They can sit and talk with the family for a few more minutes.

7. Have your children clear their plates; take turns clearing the table, and doing the dishes!

    Why should Mom (or any cook) be stuck with all of the clean up work after she cooked? Enlist help from the "troops" before they all scamper away! They need to know that the "Dish Fairy" doesn't just show up in the middle of the night.

    Teach them to rinse and put dishes right into the dishwasher so they don't pile up in the sink. Then have them unload once they are clean. It cuts down on Mom's workload, and teaches the kids responsibility within the family!

#5 – Teach your children to set the table!

Assign each child a day to set the table, and let them choose the plates, cups, napkins, placemats, etc.

If you are old enough to remember Home Economics in high school, you may have been taught how to "properly" set a table, otherwise, it's a lost art.

There's a diagram on the next page to help show where everything goes:

- The dinner plate goes in the middle.
  The edge of the plate should be set 1 inch from the edge of the table.
- The knife goes on the right of the plate, blade facing in.
- The spoon goes on the outside of the knife.
- The fork and the napkin go on the left.
- The cup or glass goes at the top of the knife.
- Don't forget the salt, pepper, and napkins for the table!

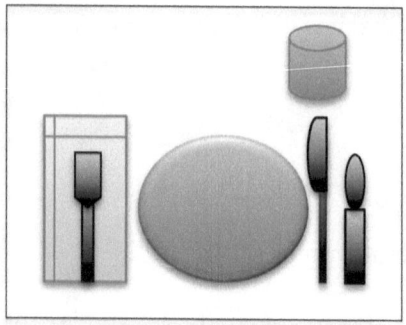

Chapter 13

A Final Thought

It is my sincere hope that you now feel inspired, challenged, encouraged, and equipped to begin to "Ditch the Drive-Thru!"

I am not telling you to NEVER go through a drive-thru, or NEVER buy fast food! I buy fast food. I didn't call it, "Never, Never, Never, Never, Never Go Through the Drive-Thru!" (That didn't fit on the business card! HA!) In fact, the decal on the back of my van reads, "Ditch the Drive-Thru!" followed by "If you're behind me in a drive-thru… I'm doing RESEARCH!" ☺

It's ok to hit the drive-thru every once in a while, but just do it ONCE in while, NOT all the time, and certainly NOT because you feel like you don't have any other option or plan. That was the main reason I added the recipes to this book!

I've had several people ask me about my culinary background, and if I am a "chef". I used to answer, "No" to that question, however now I respond with this answer: "Yes, I am a 'Chef'... I am the 'Executive Chef' of the Kennedy Kitchen!"

When this light bulb came on for me, it changed my whole outlook: I am the "Executive Chef" of MY kitchen, and I will continue to offer a nutritious menu and serve healthy meals to my family!

If you are the one doing the grocery shopping at your house, and you are the one doing the cooking for your family, then YOU are the "Executive Chef" of YOUR kitchen! (No offense to all of the "real", properly trained chefs out there!) YOU are responsible for the food that you buy, and the "menu" that you are offering to your family.

> *"YOU are the one who holds the power to help your family 'change the nutritional environment of your home'!"*

Believe me, I KNOW first hand that life is crazy, and I know how it feels to be overworked, over-tired, over-stressed, overweight, and overwhelmed!

However, I have also experienced the positive, successful results that come when I have a game plan, I choose healthier foods, and I "Get My Move On!" Now it's your turn! ☺

For your yourself, for your wallet, for your waistline, and especially for your children...

It's time to "*Ditch the Drive-Thru!*"

Blessings!

Debbi Kennedy, Founder

Additional Notes...

As you begin cooking, you may want to write down new recipes and
meal ideas. Here's a place to keep them all together!
I've also included a shopping list you can copy and take to the store!
You're welcome, and happy cooking! ☺

_____

_____

_____

_____

_____

_____

_____

_____

_____

_____

_____

_____

_____

_____

_____

_____

"Ditch the Drive-Thru!" Grocery Shopping List

Produce

- ☐ Apples
- ☐ Bananas
- ☐ Blueberries
- ☐ Grapes
- ☐ Kiwi
- ☐ Grapefruit-red
- ☐ Strawberries
- ☐ Asparagus
- ☐ Avocados
- ☐ Broccoli
- ☐ Cabbage
- ☐ Carrots
- ☐ Celery
- ☐ Garlic
- ☐ Lettuce
- ☐ Mini peppers
- ☐ Mushrooms
- ☐ Onions
- ☐ Purple potatoes
- ☐ Soy Beans
- ☐ Spinach
- ☐ Yams
- ☐ Zucchini

Meat

- ☐ Chicken
  - Thighs
  - Breasts
  - Tenderloins
- ☐ Ground Turkey
- ☐ Salmon
- ☐ Tilapia
- ☐ Boneless
  Pork Chops
- ☐ Steak
  - London Broil
- ☐ Lunch meat
  - Turkey & Ham

Dairy

- ☐ Low sugar & fat
  Greek yogurt
- ☐ Low fat cottage
  cheese
- ☐ Low fat finely
  shredded cheese
- ☐ Cheese sticks
- ☐ Large eggs
- ☐ Egg substitute
- ☐ Fru Fru Coffee
  Creamer!

Frozen Foods

- ☐ Broccoli florets
- ☐ White corn
- ☐ Petite Peas
- ☐ Mixed veggies
- ☐ Pepper strips
- ☐ Steamer bags
  - Brown rice
  - Fried rice

Canned Food & Jars

- ☐ Tuna- in water
- ☐ Chunk chicken
- ☐ Black beans
- ☐ Kidney beans
- ☐ Garbanzo beans
- ☐ Diced tomatoes
- ☐ Mandarin
  oranges
- ☐ Salsa
- ☐ Ragu Sauces
  - Garden Veggie
  - Light Alfredo
- ☐ Light Cream of
  Chicken soup

Bread & Cereal

- ☐ Low sugar,
  high fiber cereal
- ☐ Quick cook
  instant oats
- ☐ Steel cut oats
- ☐ Wheat bread
- ☐ Hot dog buns
- ☐ Low fat
  Fajita tortillas

Boxed Food

Whole grain pasta
- ☐ Spaghetti
- ☐ Linguini
- ☐ Penne
- ☐ Veggie Rotini

- ☐ Egg noodles
- ☐ Oriental Ramen

- ☐ Betty Crocker
  Super Moist Cake
  Mix - Mug Cakes!
- ☐ White Angel
  Food Cake Mix

Oil/Spices/Other

- ☐ Olive Oil
- ☐ Pure Coconut Oil
- ☐ Seasoned salt
- ☐ Garlic pepper
- ☐ Lemon pepper
- ☐ Brown sugar
- ☐ BBQ sauce
- ☐ Light Oriental
  salad dressing
- ☐ Slivered almonds
- ☐ Flax seeds